Perfectly Broken

My Life With Brittle Bone Disease and Finding Peace in the Pieces

Taniya Faulk

Perfectly Broken: My Life With Brittle Bone Disease and Finding Peace in the Pieces.

Photography and graphic design by Keith Stein of Anchor & Lace Photography

ISBN (978-0-578-34928-2)

For Mom, and for anyone who has ever felt so broken that they would permanently fall apart. I see you. I was you.

Table of contents

Foreword

In addition to being among my closest friends, I believe Taniya Faulk is among the most inspiring women to ever walk the Earth. Our friendship has grown over the past few years for a number of reasons, but I feel like one of the most significant reasons is that Taniya is one of the few people I've hardly ever heard complain. She's had as many reasons to adopt a victim mentality as anyone I know, but she never has.

We were both born with physical disabilities that make things like traveling or getting dishes off the top shelf a lot more difficult. I was born a quad amputee. My arms end at the elbows and my legs end at the knees. But the philosophy my parents raised me with was very similar to the way she was raised: focus on everything we were capable of doing and less on the things we lacked.

Don't get me wrong — she whines about little stuff. Life stuff. Work stuff. She voices her opinion openly at me for watching too much Fox News and we end up having some very spirited debates about the future of humanity. I demand that she notifies me or her neighbors before attempting to change a light bulb with a step stool. I fear that may be the most likely way we'd lose her. Hardly anything else could stop her.

I believe more than anything it's her gratitude and perspective on life that has kept her going through all of the challenges she's faced. She's able to laugh about things that would break most people in two.

She's had over a hundred broken bones. Imagine that. She's overcome a life-threatening stroke. It's hard for me to even fathom dealing with the cards she was dealt.

I wish I could have met her mother. Overcoming her loss may have been the most difficult thing she's had to endure, especially with how much her mother helped shape her. But I feel like this book is an opportunity to get as close to that as I will in this life.

I'm a believer that the little nuances of how people are raised end up having enormous effects on the rest of their lives. For me, it was little things like my grandmother taking me into grocery stores and having me practice meeting people and shaking their hands. She would always tell me that when people hear your voice and they see your face, everything else will fade away. That they'd forget about the disability entirely.

As the author of a book called *No Excuses,* I usually feel like I'm the one who needs to keep it together most of the time. However, Taniya is the friend I go to when I need to vent. She listens, but she won't let anyone in her life wallow.

Taniya has that effect on people. She may have Brittle Bone Disease, but she's one of the least frail people I know. She routinely amazes me with the way she not only figures out a way to do things physically, but also with the way she thinks. I'm confident there's still a lot I will learn from her and her journey.

My parents taught me a long time ago that everyone on the planet has a disability of some sort. Sometimes you can see them, sometimes you can't. I have no idea what your disability is. But I am pretty confident that whatever it is, you'll be able to learn something from my friend's story. I haven't had the opportunity to read beyond the introduction yet, but I know for a fact that the heart she puts into everything will be evident in these pages.

Taniya, I love you and am amazed by your heart and courage! I hope you continue to inspire many more people through this book and everywhere it takes you!

Kyle Maynard, **National Wrestling Hall of Fame, author of the New York Times Bestseller *No Excuses,* and two-time ESPY award winner**

Introduction

Growing up, my mom used to say that God has a sense of humor. I never knew what she meant by that. I had whimsical images of God sitting around telling jokes to Jesus or of him laughing at me when I did something silly. I never pictured an all-knowing deity who laughs with malice at our trials and failures. I still don't. But I do think he's found it amusing to alter my "plans" from time to time. As if to say, "Ha ha. What I have planned for you is better than anything you thought you planned!"

My life has always been marked by a series of inconvenient interruptions, whether it was a broken leg the day before I was supposed to start swim lessons or needing emergency surgery weeks before the opening night of a play I'd been the Assistant Director of. More often than not, I'd roll my eyes and silently explain to God that I had things to do, and his interruptions were not funny.

I also remember the other thing mom always said: " The quickest way to have people give up on you is to give up on yourself. The minute you quit because things don't go according to your plan is the minute you lose people's belief in you. There is no shortage of people ready to give up on you." Mom wasn't a quitter and she worked hard to make sure I wasn't either. There was no rule book to teach me how to avoid quitting. I had to be willing to adapt. I became really good at abandoning what I thought should be and embracing what was.

Having Osteogenesis Imperfecta, or Brittle Bone Disease, I found peace in letting everything fall apart and trusting that all I had to do was not quit. I had no control over if or when I would break my next bone. What I could control was how quickly I could adapt and pick up where I left off before my life was interrupted. I had to believe that the broken pieces would be stronger than before.

I don't know why I expected this book would be any different.

Maybe because I couldn't anticipate that after writing an entire book, I wouldn't be able to read it to finish editing it. Or maybe it was because I didn't know that at 41 I was going to have an Ischemic Stroke that would leave me without words.

The night started like any normal Tuesday night. I clocked out of work for the night. It felt like it had been an unusually long day. I was looking forward to settling in with a glass of red wine and some trashy reality TV. I grabbed my phone to call my best friend, Alex. She'd been my best friend since I was 15. We still speak every night. She knows me just as well as my own sister. I looked down at my phone to call her, and I couldn't read anything on it. I saw what I thought were letters, but they were all displaced. The apps made less sense than the names in the phone book. They were just one big blur of blue light. I was becoming increasingly annoyed by the phone, never thinking the problem might be with me.

Suddenly, my sister Ashley called me. Ashley is the family alarmist. She operates with so much urgency that I often wonder how her brain processes so quickly. She's also a bit of a hypochondriac. I remember when she convinced herself that she may have gotten Anthrax in the mail. I still tease her about that.

She immediately asked me, "What's wrong with you?"

I was fine. What did she mean?

"I'm fine," I told her.

"You don't sound fine," she rebuffed.

She was overly concerned, even for her. I felt perfectly normal. I was pretty certain I sounded fine. The only issue I could identify was that I was annoyed that my phone was still not working. I couldn't understand why she was being so pushy. Perhaps she was just homesick. A week earlier, Ashley had relocated to Louisiana. With 1,400 miles between us, that's the furthest we've ever lived from each other in our lives. I can't lie. I missed her too. Maybe that's why I didn't sound "fine." Maybe because I would have rather been eating dinner with her and my nieces, Gianna and Mia.

Alex finally called me. She was much more level-headed than Ashley. I was looking forward to this call; a lighthearted conversation and someone who would certainly agree that Ashley was overreacting. Almost immediately I struggled as I tried to tell her about my day. I wasn't confused. I knew what I wanted to say. The call with Ashley had just happened. I should not be having a problem recounting it, but I couldn't tell the story. Finally, Alex broke through all the "um's" and "ah's" that were littered throughout my speech.

She said, "This is about to be a really long conversation!"

At that moment, I realized that all my "um's" and "ah's" were supposed to be words—words that I couldn't make come out of my mouth. Ashley was right. I didn't sound "fine."

I knew I needed help, and I needed help now!

My dad is known for a lot of things. His speed was never one of them. Ashley and I joked that if he and a slug were in a race, the slug would win. He does not like rushing, which never made him particularly good in an emergency. Maybe that's why Ashley has such a sense of urgency—she stole his. Now that he's 67 with Emphysema, he moves even slower because he has to pace himself so he doesn't lose his breath. I know this about him. Yet I called him. It was the only three letters in my phone I could recognize: D.A.D.

"Dad, I need to go to the hospital. Something's wrong."

Alex didn't wait and had an ambulance dispatched to my house. I was taken by ambulance to the hospital. I speak for a living. I'm a writer. I've been an actress, I've starred in plays. Why was I suddenly rendered speechless? Suddenly it hit me: I WAS HAVING A STROKE. I took a graduate Neurology class. I studied the brain at length. I knew the signs and symptoms of a stroke, and I was in the middle of one. The paramedic tried to help me construct a timeline of my day in an effort to make sure it wasn't "too late."

I desperately wanted to scream, "It's not too late. I am still connected to my body. I am not dying! I just can't speak." However, those words would not come out. I heard the sirens and saw the street lights out the window as we passed them. I could hear the paramedic say over the radio, "ETA five minutes out. Patient's speech and cognition have declined during transfer."

My gut twisted when I heard him say that. *Oh, you're going to be one of them*, I thought. The players and the setting always differed, but the narrative was always the same. *She's not going to make it.* I've heard some incarnation of that my entire life.

"This poor, disabled girl who has this unforgiving disease..."

"She'll never walk..."

"This bone cannot be fixed..."

"We've done all we can..."

"College graduation won't happen. Drop out..."

What has never been included in that narrative is that Deborah Faulk did not raise a quitter. I will come out of this! I will adapt to whatever normal may look like after a stroke. Just like I adapted to every cast, wheelchair, surgery, and procedure I've lived through.

What I won't do is let another person give up on me so much that the paramedic thinks I'm willing to die in the back of this ambulance.

I was lucky. The stroke did not leave me with any loss of motor function or any real cognitive deficits. My speech returned within a day or two. I breathed a sigh of relief and was ready to move on...until I realized I couldn't read or write. I could see the words on the page, but I couldn't read them. I could identify the letters, but I couldn't put them together to form full words.

I wrote an entire book and suddenly couldn't read it to finish editing it. It would take several weeks before I regained the ability to read, write, and spell. My "planned" timeline for the completion of this book was pushed back.

Just another inconvenient interruption.

Maybe mom was right. God does have a sense of humor. She was also right when she said that there's no shortage of people ready to give up on me.

I know my life was not destined for a linear path. It's been a life filled with interruptions, "curveballs," and seemingly senseless delays. Life is rarely linear for anyone. I've never met anyone whose life was not filled with ups and downs. Moments of joy. Moments of sadness and those "interruptions" that cause you to question everything you think you know.

The masks that are the symbol of theatre—the Greek Comedy and Tragedy masks—could easily symbolize life and the human experience. I've laughed as much as I've cried. My life has been equal parts comedy and fleeting tragedy.

Genesis

I grew up being told I was *special*. It just depended on who was saying it, if being special was negative or positive.

I was the first child of my parents, Deborah and Lamont Faulk. In actuality, I was the first surviving child. My mother lost their first to a miscarriage. She didn't talk about it much, but that miscarriage impacted the way my mom would mother. Every day I knew I was wanted. Unbeknownst to me, I was branded a survivor just by being born.

My mom was the type of mother you could only dream of. She loved me and my sister fiercely. She had a turbulent childhood. She was the daughter of an abusive alcoholic mother. Like many children of alcoholics, Deborah stayed with what was familiar when picking a life partner and married an alcoholic.

Some of my earliest memories of my father are mostly of him passing out after a night of heavy drinking. My dad tried to absolve himself of the guilt by reminding us all that he only drank beer. It didn't matter if he downed twelve of them in a night. It was "only beer."

The myth of the "functional alcoholic" was so pervasive in the '80s. You could get blackout drunk every night, as long as every morning you got up and punched a clock. The world would nod in agreement that you didn't have a problem. As long as you had a job, you were somehow better than the degenerates passed out in the back of a seedy bar that got escorted home by the local police.

My parents' marriage made zero sense. They were polar opposites. My mom was a decisive and motivated woman. She had more dreams and aspirations than she had time to fill them. My dad, on the other hand, is lazy and complacent. Looking back, I know the only reason their marriage lasted as long as it did was because my mom was fiercely independent. That's where I get in from. She was determined to give my sister and me the best life possible. She knew she didn't need my dad to make that happen, so she didn't push to mold him into what she wanted him to be. Instead, she settled for what he was and made sure she was the woman who could get the job done when he faltered.

As a baby, I developed right on target. I grew at an average rate and hit every milestone right on time. I took my first steps at nine months old. There was no indication that in a few years I'd go from a happy and healthy baby to a handicapped child. No one could have known that there was a life-changing medical diagnosis about to rock my parents' idea of normal.

I remember the first day of my new normal. My sister Ashley wasn't born yet. My mother was an extremely attentive mother. She watched my every move, but I was an energetic four-year-old. The world was my playground, and I had a keen ability to sense when mom was about to focus on something else. In those rare moments, I'd seize the opportunity to explore the world around me and test boundaries. This day was no different.

Mom took me with her to the local insurance office. It was time to renew her car insurance, and dad was working. As she sat with the agent, I noticed two chairs next to each other at a nearby empty desk. Mom was preoccupied, and I was a bored four-year-old. That was certainly a recipe for disaster.

It was 1984 and the Olympics were airing. The USA gymnastics team had been all over the television. I only had a basic understanding of what gymnastics was, but I thought they were so beautiful when they performed on the balance beam and so graceful using the gymnastic rings. Mom was busy. This was the perfect moment to turn myself into a tiny gymnast. I hoisted my body between the two empty chairs and started swinging back and forth.

"Taniya, get down from there!" Mom yelled from across the room. I just kept swinging. "You are going to fall and get hurt," she bellowed.

I knowingly ignored her warnings, and suddenly I heard a snap and my right arm felt like it had become engulfed in flames. I let my tiny body fall to the ground as I just screamed in pain.

"My arm! It burns!" I wailed as my mother rushed to my side. She frantically looked for blood or any outward sign of injury. One thing was certain, I was in pain. We went to the emergency room, where I quickly told the attending physician about the fire inside my arm. He ordered an X-ray. I could tell mom thought that was unnecessary as she subtly pointed out that I didn't fall.

I can't say I blame her. It had been a long day. I, on the other hand, was in no rush to get home. I knew my acrobatic act that had now landed us in the ER for hours definitely meant that the minute we got home mom was coming for the crown jewel of my bedroom. Every time I got in trouble, mom would take my favorite Barbie doll and put her on the top shelf of her closet. If she was really mad, I wouldn't be allowed to play with Julie, my best friend who lived across the courtyard, for a couple of weeks.

She wouldn't have to. The doctor was about to deliver the punishment when he sauntered in with the freshly developed X-ray. He posted it up on the light box.

"A radius fracture at the distal end."

I had no clue what those words meant, but I'll never forget them. Whatever this doctor was about to say in English was not going to be good!

"She broke her wrist, ma'am."

Suddenly, I felt so small. I wanted to disappear as he explained he'd put my arm in a cast and that it would need to stay on for six to eight weeks. He said it would need to be kept clean and dry.

Summer had just started. That meant no running through the sprinkler with Julie, no baths. *What about my Barbie pool? Would I have to go all summer without sending Barbie and Ken for a swim?*

I could tell by how intently my mom was staring at the doctor that she was taking very copious mental notes. I left that night in my very first cast. It went from the tips of my fingers straight up to my elbow. I'd live in that cast for a full six weeks. At the time, it was the most uncomfortable thing ever. It was heavy and cumbersome. I did do my best to keep it clean and dry though, even if at one point the plaster that wrapped around my hand got covered in McDonald's Mac sauce while I tried eating a Big Mac.

Mom was never too far away with a damp paper towel to help try to keep it clean. The day I had it removed was the best day of that summer. I was terrified of the cast cutter. It looked like an oversized vacuum cleaner with a pizza cutter attached to the end of it. When the doctor turned it on, it sounded like a power saw.

What if he accidentally cut my arm off?

I stopped him the first three times he approached my arm with that thing.

Mom gently said, "Don't you want to be free?"

I did. I wanted to get wet. I wanted to move with ease. I'm right-handed, and for those six weeks, my right hand had been in this plaster prison and it was now going to be freed. I took a deep breath, knowing there was only one way out of this cast.

"Please don't cut me!" I pleaded.

He nodded and cut that cast off within seconds. I raised my arm, astonished at how light it felt. The skin was all scaly and dry. It hadn't been washed in six weeks, and it was at least two shades lighter than the rest of my body, which had been in the sun all summer. Nonetheless, it was my arm and it was free!

That freedom was short-lived.

A few weeks later, I tripped over the bedpost in my bedroom and felt that very memorable burning in my ankle. Another trip to the ER that followed the same protocol of my first ER trip. A series of X-rays revealed I had broken my ankle.

I was unwittingly on a merry-go-round that seemed to have no end. Every few weeks, a trip, fall, or just general childhood clumsiness would land me and my parents in the ER. The specifics may have been different, but it always ended in a heavy plaster cast. Some fractures were bizarre and some mundane, but they all hurt like crazy, and I was becoming used to the pain.

Somehow in between the random trips to the ER and her painstaking caring for me during fractures, mom found time to get pregnant. My little sister Ashley was born in November of 1985. Suddenly we were a family of five: two adults, two children and the chaos that followed me.

***

In the winter, mom would make me wear footie pajamas that zipped up the front. I hated those outfits. I found them hot and constricting. They are also dangerous. Mom laid Ashley on the couch. I was in awe of this little being and wanted a better look at her. I tried to use my feet to reposition myself on the couch. The plastic on the soles of the pajama feet caused my legs to slip out from under me. I hit the floor and immediately screamed out in pain. It felt as if a lightning bolt shot up my spine. I literally saw stars. My cries startled Ashley and she started crying too. It was a cacophony of sheer noise: a five-year-old screaming in pain and an infant crying in unison. Mom came rushing into the room. She didn't know who to tend to first. She scooped Ashley up in her arms. She could tell by the look on my face that we needed to go to the ER.

That was the first time I ever saw my mom panic. She didn't want to bring an infant into the ER. She didn't even like taking me. ERs can be filled with all sorts of unsavory characters.

Dad leisurely meandered into the room. He looked at me crying on the floor and took Ashley from mom's arms.

Mom quickly told him, "Taniya fell off the couch! We need to go to the hospital!"

The unspoken question "Who will watch Ashley?" hung between them. Julie's mom, Shelby, lived just across the courtyard. Mom said she was going to run and ask Shelby to sit with Ashley while they took me to the ER. Dad stood in the doorway of our living room and literally looked frozen in time holding Ashley.

I broke his spacey gaze when I cried out, "Daddy, my butt hurts!" No matter how I shifted my weight, I couldn't stop the throbbing feeling of fire that felt like it permeated both my butt cheeks.

"I know. As soon as your mom gets back, we're going to go to the hospital," he said.

As if that statement somehow summoned her, my mom came walking in through the front door with a very perplexed Shelby trailing behind her. We could tell neither of them knew what would happen next but they moved like women on a mission. Mom was far more composed now. There was always something about my mom's confidence. When she had it, so did I.

After mom gave Shelby a quick rundown of the last time Ashley had a bottle, where to find the Pampers, and where to find the phone numbers of all our family members, we were off to the hospital. I could barely walk to the car. Every time I put one foot in front of the other, I felt a surge of pain that felt like it went from my butt to my brain. The drive to the hospital wasn't any better. Every bump or sharp turn hurt as much as the initial fall. Possibly more. As my body bounced in rhythm with the uneven ground beneath us, it felt as if I was landing on rocks. An all too familiar feeling radiated across my entire lower body. That trip felt like it took forever. My dad has always been a man of few words, and in times of stress, he practically goes mute. He stoically drove to the hospital in silence.

Once we arrived at the emergency room, I was whisked off to be X-rayed. The familiar feeling of the hard metal film cassette under my butt was more than I could tolerate this time. I pleaded with the X-ray technician to just skip the X-rays altogether.

"Give me just two good pictures," he countered.

I knew only one thing: I wanted this to be over. I wanted the X-ray done, I wanted to get my cast and go home to my baby sister. I held my breath and lay there with that cold, unforgiving metal under my buttocks and lower back. When it was done, the X-ray tech emerged from behind the protective glass and helped me to my feet. A nurse came in and said she was going to take me back to the exam room. The X-ray technician smiled warmly and wished me luck.

As the nurse and I started walking through the hall, I realized she said she was taking me back to the exam room. I was never in an exam room to begin with. After we had checked in, a medical assistant took my vital signs and I was taken, alone, to be X-rayed. That realization hit me like a ton of bricks. I was alone.

Where were my parents?

Where was this nurse taking me?

We made our way through the long hallways. She asked me how I fell. I told her all about my baby sister. She seemed particularly intrigued by that fact.

"Her name is Ashley," I said.

The nurse looked visibly uncomfortable as she ushered me into the tiny exam room. I asked her where my mom and dad were. She said she didn't know but she would find out. She turned on her heels and left.

I couldn't get up on the exam table. My butt hurt even worse now since having to lie on the X-ray table. I stood confused as to what to do next. I wanted my parents. For a brief moment, I had a fleeting thought that they were intentionally avoiding me. I had caused such trouble in recent years. I wouldn't blame them if they were annoyed. Maybe they were hungry and went to get food. It had been hours since we had lunch. I was hungry. I wouldn't be mad if they went to the Burger

King down the street. I just hoped they brought me back a kid's meal, I really wanted the toy.

After what could have been a few minutes or an hour based on how much pain I was in, in walked a man wearing a long lab coat followed by a man in a suit. The man in the lab coat was easily identifiable. He was a doctor. I had seen plenty of them. The lab coat was a dead giveaway. But I wasn't sure about the guy in the suit. They both stared at me silently for a few seconds.

" I want my mom and dad!" I said. "My butt hurts."

The doctor looked intently into my eyes but didn't say anything. The man in the suit said, "Taniya, do you know the difference between the truth and a lie?"

I quickly nodded. *Of course I knew that!* My mom drilled into my head the importance of integrity and that the minute you tell a lie, you lose all integrity.

He held up a white business card and said, "If I told you this card was black, would that be the truth or a lie?"

"A lie!" I said.

He seemed to become very cautious, but continued. "You're safe, Taniya. Mommy and Daddy are all the way down the hall. You can tell us the truth. Mommy and daddy hurt you, don't they?"

I couldn't wrap my mind around what I was being asked, but the implication was enough for me to understand that my parents were in trouble.

The doctor chimed in, "Do mommy and daddy spank you?"

My mind was racing. *Spank me?* My parents barely yelled at me. I immediately came to their defense.

"What? No!"

I made the connection that these people thought my butt hurt because my parents hit me and I freaked out. I told them about slipping off the couch after trying to get a better look at Ashley, and I realized with each word, the story sounded less believable. I was in pain. I wanted my parents and felt like a liar as I tried to convince strangers to believe the truth.

Imperfect

As I heard my mom's voice coming down the hallway, I was relieved. *They hadn't left me!*

I was going to get a cast and we were going to go home. I was half right. I had broken my Coccyx bone. The tailbone is at the very base of the spine and when I landed on my butt, after slipping off the couch, I broke mine. There was no cast for that. The only cure for a broken Coccyx is time and not much sitting.

While I was by myself being X-rayed and questioned by doctors and social workers, my parents were down the hall being interrogated by Child Protective Services. They repeated the same story I told them about slipping off the couch, landing on my butt and screaming in pain. Knowing how fiery my mom is, I'm almost surprised that we got to leave as a family that night. There are two things my mom would defend to her death: her family and her integrity. One simple fall off of a couch and suddenly both were under attack. I understand why the doctors were suspicious. I was six, seemingly healthy, but every few weeks I was in the emergency room with another injury. Something didn't add up and even my mom knew it.

I spent the next six weeks healing my "broken butt," which is what we settled on calling it since I wasn't very good at saying the word Coccyx, and I found it funny that you could break your butt. Ninety percent of the time I just lied on my stomach because that was the only position that offered any relief. I was blissfully unaware of how increasingly abnormal my life was becoming. Mom pulled me out of school while I healed. The school sent a tutor and I did my school work while lying on my belly on the den couch.

My Coccyx healed and I was running and jumping again, but the joy was short-lived. A few weeks later, I sneezed and brought my hands up to my face to cover my mouth while bringing my head down to meet my hands. My right hand collided with my head and I broke my wrist.

Again, I had to fend off the implication that my parents had somehow caused this injury. I felt the burden of having to defend my parents because, at six, I couldn't control the narrative. Nothing I said fit with the story that the doctors, nurses and CPS wanted me to tell. I was torn between needing to defend my parents and trying to please the other adults. I felt trapped and helpless. Doctors asked me what happened and I told them.

"When I sneezed, my head hit my hand."

They looked at me disapprovingly. I knew they wanted a better answer, but I was raised to tell the truth.

My parents lived under this cloud of suspicion. Every emergency room visit, they wondered if this would be the time that they lost their kids and were actually charged with child abuse. I may not have fully understood, but I felt the weight of that. Every time I broke something, I felt guilty. I worried that I was somehow getting my parents in trouble. However, my next fracture would ultimately exonerate them.

Eight weeks after the sneeze that broke my wrist, all X-rays indicated that my wrist was healed. It was time to get my cast off. Like all my previous cast removals, I was super excited. I couldn't wait to get in the bathtub, wash my hands normally and just be free of the cumbersome, heavy plaster.

The doctor started sawing through the plaster with the cast cutter. I felt the vibration of the cast cutter, a sensation that I'd experienced so many times before. The cast was now cut in half and I was beaming. I couldn't wait for the freedom that was coming. I knew from experience that the doctor would use a tool to pry the two halves apart, allowing me to just lift my arm out of the remnants of plaster. That's how it was supposed to go. As the doctor started applying pressure to separate the two halves, I could feel pressure on the underside of my arm. It made me uneasy, but I was so anxious to be free of the cast that I didn't say anything. Before I knew it, I screamed. I felt the fire.

"You just broke my arm!" I told the doctor.

"No, I didn't. Your arm is healed now," the doctor assured me.

"I only feel the fire when it's broken," I explained through a steady stream of tears. "And my arm is on fire now."

To placate me, he sent me for X-rays which revealed a new Ulna fracture. The doctor stood speechless as he stared at the X-ray. *Could my bones be so brittle that the minimal pressure created by removing the cast caused a fracture?*

Nobody had a clear explanation for what had just happened. However, one thing was clear: my parents didn't do it. I left the doctor's office that day with a new cast, even though I had expected to leave with no cast at all. The doctor was still perplexed when he asked the one question that would change the course of my life forever.

"Have you taken her to see any of the specialists in the city?"

***

New York City is home to some of the most prestigious hospitals in the world. People travel from all over the country to see specialists here. Growing up on Long Island, New York City was practically my backyard. Despite how close New York City is, no doctor had ever suggested we go there looking for answers.

If there were specialists, why weren't we ever directed to them?

Mom was visibly angry. Her and dad were treated like criminals by Long Island doctors. She knew that I needed doctors and the medical community, but she also knew I needed the *right* doctors. Every few weeks, I had another broken bone and nobody had any answers. If a specialist was what I needed, mom would have moved Heaven and Earth to get me there. *Who knew there were specialists besides the orthopedist I had already seen?*

She was frustrated with the cycle of breaking a bone, getting a cast, removing the cast and breaking something else so we could start over. She witnessed most of my fractures. They weren't the result of clumsiness or some major physical trauma. There was something different about me and we all knew it. The question was exactly how different? And why? With those lingering questions. We were officially New York City-bound.

The first stop was The Hospital for Special Surgery. There, I met an orthopedic surgeon, Dr. John Healey. He didn't look like a doctor. He didn't have graying hair and a pot belly like other doctors I'd seen. *Maybe doctors in New York City just look different?*

Dr. Healey wasn't an ordinary orthopedic surgeon. He specialized in rare bone conditions. Mom showed up with X-rays compiled like an artist's portfolio and every detail she could remember about the first six years of my life. Dr. Healey listened intently as she told him about the broken wrist in the insurance office, followed by the broken ankle a few weeks later, another broken wrist, my broken butt and yet another broken wrist. He was seemingly mesmerized by my eyes. He kept looking in them with his pen light.

"Blue Sclera present," he announced without further context.

My parents looked at each other, mentally asking each other, "What the hell does that mean?"

Dr. Healey went on to explain a really rare disease: Osteogenesis Imperfecta. He said that it only affects one in every 100,000 live births. The defining characteristic was bones that break with little to no stress. Patients with the disease also have a distinct blueish tint to the whites of their eyes known as Blue Sclera. I was always complimented on my very intense and unique eyes.

Dad stared blankly while mom took copious notes.

Osteogenesis Imperfecta is a genetic disorder that inhibits the body's ability to produce sufficient collagen. This results in an array of problems with connective tissue, most notably within the musculoskeletal system. Today, there are several different types of the disease that have been discovered which vary in severity. They all have a single common denominator: extreme bone fragility.

In 1986, Dr. Healey knew about two types: Osteogenesis Imperfecta Congenita, meaning it was present at birth and some fractures occurred in utero, or Osteogenesis Imperfecta Tarda, which was not present at birth and often fractures did not begin until the child began weight-bearing. I fell into the latter category.

Outside of having a fancy name for what was wrong with me, the actual diagnosis didn't change much. Dr. Healey was forthcoming in his assertion that there was no known cure and there was no medication I could take to strengthen my bones. My parents had more questions than there were answers.

If this thing was genetic, how did I get it since neither one of them had it?

What about Ashley? Would she have it?

Genetics and genealogy were still in their infancy in the late 1980s. There wasn't a genetic test for Osteogenesis Imperfecta, OI for short.

However, Dr. Healey sent my parents to meet with a geneticist. Using a family tree that my mom supplied and a rundown of our family history, the geneticist determined that OI was not present in the last six generations on either side of my family. She deemed that my diagnosis was the result of a "spontaneous genetic mutation." There was no indication that Ashley had it. Although no one could be sure because she was still a baby, and she wasn't mobile yet. When I was a baby, I was happy and healthy too!

It was as if getting the diagnosis opened the flood gates. I started to get fractures more often. Some days, simply getting out of bed was enough to cause a fracture. One morning, I stood up and felt my ankle crack underneath me before falling to the ground. As if on cue, mom rushed into the bedroom as I let out that telltale scream.

"My ankle's broken," I told her.

I didn't need an X-ray to know. I was so familiar with the sound the bone makes as it breaks and that intense feeling of the limb being on fire. I was diagnosing my own fractures before we even made it to the emergency room. The X-rays would later confirm what I already knew.

Well-meaning family and friends would try to force me to drink more milk. I loathed milk. The smell, the viscosity and the fact that people wanted me to drink it was enough to turn my stomach. I was growing up in the '80s. If the decade had a catchphrase, it was, "Got milk?" Even Saturday morning cartoons were interrupted by multiple milk commercials normally consisting of some healthy-looking white boy running and jumping and then morphing into an adult flexing his muscles. The message was clear as day: you want an active lifestyle? You want to be healthy and strong? You better pour yourself a nice cold glass of milk. I wanted all of those things so the advertising dollars were not lost on me, but I hated milk. Even mom jumped on the "Got milk?" bandwagon. She made sure there was always chocolate and strawberry syrup in the fridge so I'd reluctantly take my glass of milk. Somehow, she thought I would find pink strawberry-flavored milk less disgusting than milk-flavored milk. Mom didn't like milk either so she didn't push it too much. There wasn't then, nor is there now, any evidence that drinking milk would have any impact on my fracture rate.

***

When Ashley was a toddler learning to walk, there was poetic irony in that. I couldn't stand without my legs crumbling beneath me as my baby sister was learning how to walk. Like any toddler, she fell down, and she fell often. Every time she would fall, mom would hold her breath, and she wouldn't exhale until she was able to pick Ashley up and check her for injuries. She was always okay, and mom would sigh with relief and put her down. I was sitting on the floor while Ashley was cruising around our coffee table. I watched her in awe. In a moment of bravery, she let go of the coffee table. She swayed back and forth briefly before she lost her balance and plopped down on my right leg. She weighed all of 20 pounds and didn't fall from some great height. It should have been an uneventful fall, but I have OI.

My femur broke.

I felt the tears flood my face as I screamed for mom, who was in the kitchen making sandwiches. Poor mom looked so confused when she walked in. I was crying and Ashley was crying. If you hadn't seen the fall, you wouldn't know anything was wrong. It appeared as if Ashley was just sitting on my lap. I had my arms wrapped around her and pressed my face into her back.

"She broke my leg," I stammered.

I couldn't understand why I got hurt when Ashley was the one who fell.

That was the first time it occurred to me that Ashley and I would have very different lives. Not necessarily better or worse, but different. Even something as universal as gravity treated my body differently than it treated hers. It was official: I was fragile but would need to become tough as nails.

Dad was at work, so mom's only option was to call an ambulance. I couldn't walk on my leg. There was no way she could carry me, stabilize my broken femur and carry a toddler. I liked ambulances.

The rides always felt less bumpy than the rides we took in Dad's old Buick. I thought it was exciting that ambulances could "break the rules." I'd giggle with delight as they'd race through red lights with the sirens blaring. The downside to taking the ambulance was that it was going to take me to the nearest hospital. I was going to be seen by whatever on-call orthopedic surgeon was working in the ER. I wasn't going to be seen by Dr. Healey. That was frightening. To date, Dr. Healey had been the only doctor with any plausible theories as to what I had.

When we got to the emergency room, mom was immediately on defense.

The doctor simply asked, "What happened?" He literally just meant, "What brings you to the Emergency Room tonight?"

"She has Osteogenesis Imperfecta," mom emphatically announced and launched into a full-blown monologue about how I am Dr. Healey's patient at The Hospital for Special Surgery.

Essentially my mom was name-dropping. She was putting this doctor on notice that I had a doctor, I had a diagnosis and she was not a child abuser. He looked at her for a moment as she stared back at him. He admitted that he didn't have much experience with OI, but ordered an X-ray. After all, a broken bone is a broken bone, and the best way to diagnose that is with an X-ray.

When the film came back, he slapped it up on the light box and immediately zeroed in on a stark white line on the film across the femur bone. "Yea, she broke her femur."

I nodded in agreement. He then pointed to the four or five other faint lines that littered the image.

"Actually, it looks like she broke her femur several times."

Any semblance of composure mom had, she just lost it at this point.

"Yes! I told you, she has Osteogenesis Imperfecta. You know, Brittle Bone Disease!"

If looks could kill, that doctor was about to be six feet under. Trying to calm her, he coolly said, "Yes, you did say that. I'm not all that familiar with that disease."

Things would have been okay if he stopped there, but he wanted to keep talking. As if he wanted it known that he had some knowledge. He had to say something;

"What I do know is these kids tend not to live very long."

My mom's face changed. She no longer looked angry and defensive, she looked incredibly sad. I wasn't affected by what he said as much as I was by how sad it seemed to make my mom feel. She didn't push him on what he meant by that. If I weren't within earshot or if she could have asked me to leave, I'm sure she would have asked him.

Mom had a saying: "Opinions are like assholes. Everybody has one." I know she wanted to believe the idea that a short life expectancy was just the opinion of some small-town doctor with zero experience treating patients with my disease. However, I could instantly tell it worried her.

The Glass Doll

Every few weeks, we'd make the trip from Long Island to New York City for follow-up appointments with Dr. Healey. The cast for my femur fracture went all the way up my entire leg. I couldn't sit up in the backseat of the car so my parents rented a van for every trip so I could lay comfortably across the backseat. I loved those trips. My favorite part was when we got to go through the Midtown Tunnel. The Midtown Tunnel takes drivers from Queens straight into Midtown Manhattan, but it does so underwater. Driving through it, you'd never know that you are driving under the East River. That tunnel takes you from where you are to where you want to be, perfectly protected from the unpredictable river waters that surround you. In many ways, that tunnel was a metaphor for my early childhood. I was always underwater but protected and insulated by the adults in my life, mainly my mom. Without that insulation, I couldn't have moved through my earliest years of life.

Dr. Healey was seemingly unfazed by my most recent femur fracture. It was a straightforward fracture and would heal. It also had a cause: Ashley fell on me. He was more concerned with the fractures that were occurring without cause. It was clear that weight-bearing was no longer healthy for me. Simply standing placed too much stress on my legs, and they literally would fracture beneath me. He reviewed my most recent femur X-ray and noted all the small previously healed fractures on there. He had me come back for a series of X-rays on both legs, suspecting I'd had more fractures than we knew about. Sure enough, those X-rays showed many healed fractures up and down my legs. Mainly femur fractures, but the tibias and fibulas had also broken more times than we treated.

They're called stress fractures—tiny cracks from repeated stress on the bone. Stress fractures are common in athletes because of the repeated force imposed on their bodies by physical activity. In kids like me, stress fractures occur by simply shifting my weight from one leg to the other, sitting on a toilet that is too hard, or rolling over in bed too quickly. These were fractures I didn't identify as fractures. There was no fire, no tears, and no trips to the emergency room. I'd tell mom my leg hurts, limped when I walked for a few weeks and that was the end of it. Despite how uneventful they seemed, they were still fractures. Stress fractures can open and become bigger, more problematic fractures, though.

Maybe the writing was on the wall the entire time, and Dr. Healey finally decided to say it. He suggested I should stop walking. *How would that work? What were the alternatives to walking?* I wondered at the time.

He wanted me to get fitted for a wheelchair. I know this made sense to him from a medical perspective. But to me, it made no sense. I could walk, run, jump, and climb. *Why should I use a wheelchair?*

Sure, after six or eight weeks in a cast, the muscle atrophy would be severe and it would take months for me to regain function, only to fracture again. I was in this vicious cycle that didn't seem like it was going to let up anytime soon. Limiting my fractures meant limiting my pain and reducing muscle atrophy and loss of function. To increase my function, he wanted to limit my mobility.

As a little kid, one of the only things you have complete control over is how you move. *Do I walk or do I run? Do I feel like skipping or hopping through the playground?* I was being told I had to give that up. Two years earlier, I was a hyper four-year-old, running and jumping. Suddenly I was being told that just walking was dangerous.

Dr. Healey dubbed me "The glass doll." He encouraged my parents to carry me on a pillow. My dad already did a considerable amount of carrying me. For example, whenever I broke my leg, I was rendered completely immobile. Doctors never offered me crutches. I'll never know if that was just a sign of the times. Perhaps in the '80s they didn't give kids crutches as freely as they hand them out today. I think it's more likely that every doctor that treated me just recognized my innate clumsiness and knew asking me to balance on a set of crutches with the added weight of a heavy plaster cast was a disaster waiting to happen. Dad would dutifully carry me wherever I needed to go. Although, most of my time during leg fracture healing was spent lying on the couch.

The prospect of not being able to walk ever again weighed heavily on me. I didn't talk about it. I wish I had because I thought about it all the time. I knew I wasn't like other kids, but I *felt* like other kids. I felt *normal*. Running and jumping were a part of that normalization. It wasn't using a wheelchair that bothered me. It was everything that I assumed was about to be taken away from me. I didn't actually know anyone who used a wheelchair, but I distinctly remembered the first time I saw someone in a wheelchair.

***

The year before, mom and dad took me to the mall to get my ears pierced for my fifth birthday. I was so excited. I wanted my ears pierced like mom's. I had a broken wrist so I was relegated to safe activities for my birthday. When dad offered me the opportunity to get my ears pierced, I jumped at the chance. We went to a little kiosk near the food court. I picked out a pair of heart-shaped ruby studs. Red was my favorite color. Dad picked me up and put me in the oversized chair. Two girls approached me, each carrying a piercing gun. I watched as one girl opened my new heart-shaped ruby studs. She handed one to the other girl who had made her way to the other side of me. They each loaded an earring in their respective piercing gun. It dawned on me at that moment that in order to get these pretty red studs in my ears, I needed holes in my earlobes! I knew I didn't come to the mall with holes in my earlobes, and I panicked.

"Is this going to hurt?" I asked.

I was sitting on a chair with a broken wrist. My twentieth broken bone in a year, and I wanted to know if an ear piercing was going to hurt. The irony of that was not lost on my parents, who both chuckled.

"Oh, you'll just feel a little pinch," one of the girls said as she quickly looked away.

In my mind, that phrase will go down in history as the biggest lie adults tell to children. She marked the spot that would be pierced with an X, and as if on cue, both girls positioned their piercing guns and started the slowest count to three ever.

"One."

I took a deep breath.

"Two."

I took three deep breaths.

"Three"

They simultaneously pulled their triggers and my new heart-shaped ruby studs were thrust through my earlobes. I cried uncontrollably. One of the girls quickly grabbed a handheld mirror and shoved it in my face so I could see my new earrings. My earlobes were almost as red as the ruby hearts, my eyes were puffy and my face was flushed. I had cried a lot out of pain in my life, but this was the first time I had ever seen myself cry. I was oddly intrigued by my own reflection. I was a little brown girl whose cheeks were becoming red. My bottom lip was quivering. My shirt was wet with my own tears. I wondered if this is what I looked like every time I walked into the emergency room crying because I broke something. It was the first time I got to feel minor pain. No fire inside the broken limb, no screaming. Just simple soreness that would resolve in a few hours. There was also a reward for the pain: new sparkly earrings. As we walked through the mall, I looked at my reflection in the glass windows of every store we passed. I don't know what I expected to see, but I made it a point to look.

As we approached one of the large department stores, I saw a woman who appeared to be sitting down inside. When I got closer to the display window, I could see she wasn't sitting in a regular chair. Her chair had four wheels. I looked past my own reflection to look at her. Suddenly I didn't care how I looked with my new earrings. In a moment of great cosmic synchronicity, I was drawn to this woman I had never met. I stared at her until she eventually rolled away. I know my stare made her uncomfortable. To this day, her image has stuck with me. My past and future merged for a split second, only separated by a display window.

When it was time to get my femur cast off, I just knew I could convince Dr. Healey that I didn't need a wheelchair. In my head, I was fully prepared to jump, do a high kick, maybe a little dance. I naively thought that if I could prove I had the strength to stand and could move my legs without breaking anything, he'd see my bones had strengthened and take the wheelchair option off the table. At six, I had no concept of just how unrealistic that expectation was. He sawed off the cast and pried it open.

So far, so good. My thigh was ridiculously thin. It was at least half its original size. My muscle had atrophied that much. He wanted me to try standing up. *It's time to do all of the silly things I used to do before my fractures became so frequent: jump up and down, do that dance I made up when I was pretending to be a tap dancer, stretch my legs behind my head, one on each side and wave at people with my feet.*

Dad hated that one. I loved making him squirm just by showing off how flexible I was. I remembered all the tricks and gymnastics that I had performed at this very moment. If Dr. Healey could see who I was before fractures, he'd know I could be that again and not need a wheelchair. In those daydreams, I lost track of reality. I was still fragile. I had a freshly healed fracture. I still had Osteogenesis Imperfecta! I scanned the room and realized just how high the exam table was. When we first walked in, my entire leg was in a cast. Dad carried me and gently placed me on the table. Looking around, it felt like I was closer to the sky than the floor. I was more than reluctant. I was downright scared to jump off the exam table.

What if I fall and fracture everything?

What if I am lucky enough to land on my feet but break both legs in the process?

Maybe I was taking too long, or maybe he saw the trepidation in my eyes, but Dr. Healey picked me up and placed me in a tiny chair. It had a nice cushion, so I knew my legs were safe from fracturing. My legs dangled off the edge, not touching the floor. Dr. Healey steadied himself on a stool with wheels and rolled over, stopping right in front of me. This was the first time we were eye to eye. Normally I was on the exam table while he towered over me. He put out his arms and asked me to stand. His voice was steady and calm. He had picked me up many times before, so I knew his arms were strong enough to catch me if I lost my balance. Yet, I kept thinking of everything that could go wrong.

What if my femur wasn't ready?

What if it broke when I stood?

I just got my cast off. I didn't want to end up back in one.

Mom and dad stood across the room with wide eyes looking at me. I knew they remembered all the things I used to do before everyone worried that I would fracture something. I wasn't a different person, but my life was drastically different. I looked at Dr. Healey's outstretched arms and tried to will my legs to stand. Everyone in that room, even the doctor, believed I could. Yet, this visceral fear took over. I was terrified and I didn't even want to try. So I didn't.

"I can't do it!" I said, my voice breaking.

A chorus of "Yes, you can," and "Just try, Tee," came from mom and dad in the doorway.

I was so afraid to stand, but I was even more afraid of letting mom or dad down and giving up. I stood up. Immediately I felt my leg quiver beneath me, and within three seconds, I collapsed into Dr. Healey's arms. More out of fear than out of fatigue. I just couldn't do it. With tears in my eyes, I apologized to mom and dad. I apologized to Dr. Healey. That is the first time I recall feeling like I failed. More than three decades later, I still wonder how different the trajectory of my life would have been had I not given into fear and just stood up. The truth is, it probably would have made no difference. My leg was atrophied and weak. I didn't give up. Physically, I was not able to stand for any significant duration of time. I needed physical therapy. I needed to be stronger. My legs just weren't ready.

Mom asked Dr. Healey about that ominous prediction made by the orthopedic surgeon who set my most recent femur fracture. Dr. Healey was the closest thing she had to an expert in my condition. If anyone was going to know if my life expectancy was going to be compromised, he would. He was noncommittal in his answer.

He shook his head, neither in agreement nor disagreement. "There's not a lot of literature on the subject," he said, as if to make his next statement a little more neutral. "Kids are resilient. They overcome more than you or I could. She could certainly beat the odds. This is a complex disease. In my experience, OI kids don't live past ten." He told her.

I quickly counted on my fingers. Ten was only four years away. I was looking forward to ten. I couldn't wait to be double digits. *Was that going to be it? Was I going to turn ten and have my life just stop?*

I knew about death and Heaven, but in my mind, dying only happened to old people. I'd never been to a funeral. I hadn't even had a pet die, but I knew death meant the end. It meant you weren't here anymore. You wouldn't get to be with your family. *Did I only have four more years to be with mom, dad and Ashley?*

In reality, Dr. Healey's words didn't actually change anything. Those four years were going to pass regardless. I was going to have this disease regardless. As a family, we were going to navigate it. Win, lose or draw, we didn't know what the future was going to hold, but mom was committed to my life in every moment that followed.

***

Shortly after that visit, I got my first wheelchair. It was candy apple red. At the time, red was my favorite color, so that was enough to thrill me. It was also bulky and heavy. Having a wheelchair did the opposite of everything I feared. I got to spend more time outside in the courtyard of our apartment complex. I could still chase Julie around and play tag with her. I couldn't jump rope, and I couldn't skate, but I was just as active as ever. I was like any other six-year-old girl, only different. I didn't use the wheelchair inside our apartment, though. It was a manual wheelchair and it was incredibly hard to maneuver on carpets. It didn't fit through the narrow doorways inside the apartment either. I preferred just being on the floor. I would scoot around on my butt. It was easy for me to get around like that, and it was safe. I was already on the floor. I liked the freedom of being unencumbered by my wheelchair, and the apartment was the only place I could do that.

***

Despite the wheelchair, my fractures seemed to become more frequent with every passing day. My life was nearly unrecognizable from the one I had at four or five. Mom withdrew me from school. I kept missing so much of it because of my injuries, that it made sense to just keep me home. If nothing else, it was safer. Even with a wheelchair for mobility, I couldn't be protected from a class full of rowdy first graders. The school sent a tutor to my home to teach me. She came in the afternoons. We'd do math, reading and practice my writing. Writing was a major task when my right arm was in a cast. It's nearly impossible to hold a pencil while a thick piece of plaster is between my thumb and index finger. I slowly became ambidextrous. When my right arm was in a cast, I learned to write with my left hand. It wasn't perfect penmanship, but it was legible. Learning in the confines and safety of my home meant my physical health was protected. Nobody considered my mental health.

I was loved…

I was cared for…

I also had no friends because I rarely saw anyone outside of my family.

Nobody meant for me to feel lonely. Loneliness was a byproduct of caution and safety.

As I grew, it was becoming clear that the bones in my legs and arms were bowed. My femurs were deformed by some poor fracture healing but also had signs of bowing, which is common for kids with OI. Dr. Healy recommended my parents consider *rodding* my long bones. Rodding is a surgical procedure in which titanium rods are inserted into the center of the bone. The goal is to prevent further bowing. During growth, it would also strengthen those bones from the inside.

Theoretically, that would slow the rate at which I would fracture. It would be an intense surgery with a lengthy recovery. He proposed I have my legs rodded first. My femurs showed the most bowing. My legs were also what broke most often. He said if rodding my legs worked out, then we could do my arms as well. I wouldn't be *cured,* but fewer fractures definitely sounded appealing.

Mom thought it sounded barbaric since rodding meant a doctor would cut me open and physically install metal rods inside bones that weren't currently broken. And it was all elective. *Who would elect to do such a thing? Who would elect to put a child through such a thing?*

It was presented as an option. A choice. However, there was no choice. If I didn't get rodded, my legs would continue to fracture consistently. They would continue to bow, and eventually, walking again would not be an option. Dr. Healy told mom and dad my best chance for ever being able to walk was to have my legs rodded and have them rodded young.

***

Dad was never a great decision-maker. The simplest of questions, such as "What do you want for dinner?" or "What should we get your mom for Christmas?" were responded to with a sigh and "Whatever you want, Deb."

When it came to Ashley, he'd give his input and consult with my mom, but he'd never give the final Okay. If things didn't go as planned, he didn't want to be the one who was blamed.

The truth is that mom liked it that way. She ran our house like a well-oiled machine and thrived under pressure. Dad could barely think if he was under too much pressure. Despite this, or maybe because of it, I know they supported each other. Mom knew dad often doubted himself, so she never pushed him into decision-making.

Even with mom at the helm, I don't know how they navigated through those early years. She was a young mother with two daughters, one of whom she wasn't even sure would live past ten years old. She was blindly making decisions. There was very little research or data on OI. Even the doctors didn't really know what they were dealing with yet. Google hadn't been invented at the time so she couldn't do countless hours of research while Ashley and I were asleep. She had to hear what the doctors were saying and make all her decisions based on what her gut told her was best. She wanted me to live, but my mom fiercely valued quality of life.

***

My rodding surgery took place in 1987 when New York City was in the grip of the AIDS epidemic. Originally believed to only affect gay men, HIV and AIDS quickly started making their way through New York City hospitals. There was a very palpable fear that resonated throughout Manhattan hospitals during those days. Hospitals all but halted the use of blood products from the New York Blood Bank, as they had discovered virus transmission to patients who received blood products. Children my age, most notably Ryan White and Joey DiPaolo, had contracted HIV simply by receiving a blood transfusion. My medical team asked my parents to donate blood that would be reserved for me should I need a transfusion during or after surgery.

I don't think you ever forget your first surgery. I was only seven years old and didn't truly understand what it meant to have surgery.

"You'll go to sleep, and while you're sleeping, we are going to make your legs stronger," my surgical team explained.

It sounded nice and whimsical, like a superhero movie. I just fall asleep, and while I'm sleeping, I get extra strength. *What would my legs look like? Would they be bigger? Would they be thicker than my current skinny legs? Or would they look like robot legs?* I knew they were going to put rods made of metal in my legs. That sounded like robot legs.

I lay on the stretcher as mom and dad both told me they loved me. They were permitted to walk alongside the stretcher as we made our way to the operating room. Each hallway seemed a little colder than the one before. At the hall leading to an oversized set of double doors, mom and dad were told they had to leave me. Dad kissed my forehead and told me he loved me. Mom lifted my hand to her lips and kissed it.

"I will be right here when you wake up," she said.

The big double doors swung open and I was pushed into the operating room. It was ice cold in there, and the lights were brighter than I had ever seen in my life.

How am I going to sleep in here under all these bright lights?

The surgical team carefully moved me from the stretcher to the actual operating table. I felt nervous as I was moved from the semi-firm mattress of the stretcher to the cold hard steel of the operating table. A nurse quickly buckled a safety belt across my abdomen. The anesthesiologists approached me, holding a mask. I could hear the oxygen hiss as it flowed through it.

"I'm going to put this mask on you and give you a little air that will make you sleepy," he said.

I wasn't sleepy. I didn't understand how air was going to make me sleepy. I felt wide awake. Even if I wasn't, the lights and all the commotion in the room were going to keep me up. Nurses and doctors were milling around me, and machines beeped and hissed next to me.

"There's medicine in this air that will make you sleepy, " he said. "All you have to do is lie there and breathe."

I looked at the mask nervously and back at the anesthesiologist.

"Think about your favorite ice cream flavor. Think about it with all the toppings you like. You'll fall asleep, and when you wake up, it will be there."

Pistachio with hot fudge. That was always my favorite. *If, after sleeping, I was going to wake up with robot legs and an ice cream sundae, then maybe I should try and fall asleep.*

He placed the anesthesia mask over my nose and mouth. I was caught off guard by how sweet the gas flowing into my nose and mouth tasted. It wasn't sweet like candy. It was sweet like the taste stamps left in your mouth after licking them. It was downright nauseating. I tried focusing on the pistachio ice cream with hot fudge that I wanted when I woke up, but nothing could take my mind off the thick, sweet-tasting gas I was breathing in. It felt like an eternity, but I drifted to sleep effortlessly.

The surgery itself took several hours. Dr. Healey rodded both femurs and tibias. I woke up in a Spica cast. In the '80s, they were simply known as body casts. It stretched from just above my belly button, ran the length of both legs and ended at my toes. A strategically placed square was cut out in the crotch to allow me to use the bathroom. It was impossible to sit up in that, so once again, I would spend months lying down. Typically used for severe femur and pelvic fractures, it is designed to keep the bones from the waist down completely immobile. Because my femurs and tibias were rodded, both legs had to be completely immobile. There was a bar made out of plaster between my legs that mom and dad could use as a handle while carrying me. The recovery was arduous. When planning the surgery, we were told I would be in a Spica cast for eight to ten weeks, but I think we were all unprepared for what that actually meant.

The cast was hot, itchy and heavy. I couldn't sit up because of how far up my torso the cast went. I'd had plenty of casts before, but this was the first time 75% of my body was encased in plaster. I was nothing short of miserable. I vacillated between being depressed and angry. There I was, just lying on the couch, a virtual prisoner while everyone moved around me. I longed to go out. A simple trip to the grocery store with mom would have been a welcomed outing.

Thank goodness for Nana and her trusty Scrabble board. My Nana was my saving grace in my early years.

Nana was this beautiful statuesque woman who I looked up to literally and figuratively. She had raised my father and his two siblings as a single mother in the '50s. There was a power and fierceness in Nana that she tempered perfectly with grace and humility. She was one of my very first models for what independence truly looked like.

Nana was also a highly skilled Scrabble player. At least once a day, she'd pull out her wooden Scrabble board and set it up on the coffee table. The anticipation I'd feel as she opened the maroon velvet bag that held the tiles is one of my greatest childhood memories. Nana was competitive. She played to win. She wasn't going to throw a game just so I could win. After playing a word, she looked it up in her pocket dictionary and read me the definition. When I'd play a word that earned me more than just a few points, she'd leap to her feet in excitement and shout, "Hot diggity dog!"

I may not have been in school, but I was becoming quite a wordsmith. I knew at least five different words that started with Q. Occasionally I'd play a word that was a bone: tibia, femur and ulna. Nana would always challenge it. She'd look it up in her pocket dictionary and read the definition. She'd realize it was a bone, and I'd tell exactly which fracture it was and how it happened.

"Remember when mom told you I broke my wrist? That was actually my ulna!" I'd quip.

Nana would smile, impressed, and I would feel smart. Nana was the first person to tell me I should be a doctor. I saw more doctors than I saw teachers. I absorbed the terminology. It was like knowing a secret code. Nana and I would play Scrabble for hours, and she would build me up, calling me smart and advanced. Since I wasn't in school, I had no measurement for success or intelligence, and whether she knew it or not, she was laying the foundation upon which all my academic success would be built. I don't know how she had the foresight to know the educational system would spend the next ten years of my life tearing me down and filling me with self-doubt. Without knowing it, Nana planted the seed of confidence in me that I would need to get through the years ahead.

***

The plan was that once I was fully rodded, I could return to school. My bones shouldn't break as easily, and if I did fracture one, it would stay in perfect alignment. I'd had displaced fractures before where the bones and the pieces of bone don't stay aligned. Those were so much more difficult to cast and took much longer to heal. A fractured bone with a rod in it can't move. They are easier to cast and would heal quicker.

I held on to the hope of going to school. That was my biggest dream. I was in the Spica cast for almost three months. The day it came off and I sat in my wheelchair again, I felt liberated. I was given back the tiny sliver of independence I had and I loved it! Even as a little kid, I hated depending on people. The fire of independence burned deep within me for as long as I can remember.

The rods seemed to be doing their intended job. My legs broke far less frequently, and when they did, it was only a minor fracture that would heal in a four- to six-week period. I was now going months between breaks. Regardless, dad was still tense and nervous around me. With each new fracture, we were driven further apart. He showed no physical affection towards me. I started to feel like he couldn't even stand to be near me. One day, I was sitting on the couch in our den while Ashley was playing on the floor. Mom called dad to join us. I wasn't sure why mom felt the need to convene the whole family, but she did. Mom did this from time to time: her unofficial family meetings. Most of the time, she would say something of little importance: a speech about keeping the house clean or questions about what we wanted as a side dish for the pork chops she was making for dinner. I think, in reality, she just wanted to see her whole family in one space. Dad was always the last one in the room when mom called. He'd be caught up in some TV show and wait until the commercial break to walk away from the TV. Whenever dad had to be called two or three times, mom would joke, "Girls, your father needs a personal invitation." We'd all laugh. Even dad.

I don't think dad wanted to be absent. He just didn't know how to be present. Mom and dad had very different childhoods. Mom's parents were happily married and were until the day they died. Dad's parents divorced when he was young. Nana held down their household when he was a kid. His dad came over for the "fun" stuff. Mom was giving dad a life that looked like the one he remembered. He could easily do "fun" stuff: Donald Duck voices at dinner, pretending to really eat the cakes made in the easy bake oven and buying candy. Dad struggled with a lot of the adult stuff, so he just avoided most of it altogether.

He finally meandered into the living room to join us for mom's meeting. I saw him in the doorway. He looked at me and the open seat next to me on the couch, and sat on the floor.

"Dad, you can sit here," I said as I indicated the spot next to me.

"No, I'm fine," he said as he shrugged casually.

My own father couldn't even bring himself to sit next to me. It was fear. He was terrified of touching me. He didn't want to be the reason I fractured. All he knew was that I had this disease that made me fragile. No one knew how much physical pressure I could take before something fractured.

What hug would be the one that broke a rib? Would a reassuring pat on the back break my shoulder blade?

It could.

These were very real possibilities. It was a risk dad wasn't willing to take. He meant it as a precautionary measure intended to keep me in one piece. I interpreted it as disdain, especially since he showered Ashley with affection. There was no shortage of hugs, kisses and roughhousing with dad for her. Looking back, that is probably the genesis of some of the animosity I would develop towards my sister in early adulthood.

School Daze

Somewhere between the planning of my rodding and the actual recovery, every well-meaning doctor and social worker got in my mom's ear about my going to school. Mom was my fiercest advocate. She wanted the absolute best for me. She had all the same hopes and dreams for me as any parent has for their child. She was also navigating uncharted territory with no guidance. There were no disabled people in our inner circle. Outside of the hospital, I don't think we ever saw disabled children. She had a small family and a handful of friends, all with varying opinions about my life and what was *best*. She fielded unsolicited suggestions to make her life easier. Her own brother told her that she should consider institutionalizing me so I don't blame her for trusting the *professionals* who recommended sending me to a school for children with disabilities. At the time, it made sense. I'd be able to receive physical therapy during my school day. There was no question if the school would be accessible for my wheelchair. I would spend the day in class with kids who looked like me. Certainly, that would be good for my self-esteem. Most importantly, I'd get my education.

Except I wouldn't.

BOCES was a school not far from my home for children with physical, emotional and learning disabilities—a hard emphasis on the learning disabilities. When I first started, I was intrigued by all the different disabilities. There were plenty of wheelchair users like me. There were also kids with walkers and crutches. I got the immediate sense that this was supposed to feel inclusive to me, but it didn't. It felt strange and foreign.

BOCES didn't look like the rest of the world. The only non-disabled people were the teachers themselves. Separating me from non-disabled children didn't make me feel more normal. In fact, it made me feel less normal. I felt less intelligent, less important and far less capable than my non-disabled peers. I knew I was in a *special* school and therefore was an *other*. That plagued my psyche. I felt just like everybody else. I knew I didn't look or move like everybody else, but I couldn't reconcile why I shouldn't be given the chance to learn like everybody else.

At school, classes were often interrupted by an outburst of one of the students who struggled with emotional control. The focus at BOCES always felt more about physical rehabilitation and less about actual education. I spent more time receiving physical therapy than I did actually being educated. The education I did receive was laughable at best. There was no differentiation between the curriculum if you were a student with an intellectual disability or a student with a physical disability. We all colored the same pictures, read the same stories and did the same worksheets.

I hated going to school. I wasn't being challenged by the work. I was bored. My wheelchair had no bearing on what I could or couldn't comprehend. Yet, here was this *special* school offering a one-size-fits-all education. I wanted out. I knew I should be grateful that I was in school. I also knew I didn't want a watered-down version of what school should be: a place to learn, grow and experience some independence. At BOCES, none of that was happening. I was stifled and felt less independent at school than I did at home. Eventually, mom got sick of seeing another picture I had colored. I'd be gone for eight hours a day, five days a week, and the most *work* I'd have to show is something I had colored.

I was lucky that I had done kindergarten in a *real* school and had learned to read during my time with a tutor. I immersed myself in books. Mom was an avid reader. There was no shortage of books around my house. Without any real homework or material to study, I'd come home from school and read anything I could get my hands on. I begged my mom to let me go to a different school. Sometimes I'd come home in tears. I was so frustrated by what I told mom was baby work.

I always had an insatiable yearning for knowledge. I questioned things most kids my age never thought about. *How did stars get in the sky? Why did the ocean move? Where did the sun go when it set?* Part of me believed that I'd learn these answers in a *real school.* A bigger part of me understood that I was being underestimated. I was too young to know what biases were, but it's as if I innately understood that all of the things I was capable of were dismissed because of the one thing I couldn't do: walk. The world viewed me as inferior. Even at eight years old, I could feel how unfair that was.

After two years of minimal educational progress, mom decided to pull me out of BOCES and enroll me in public school. It wasn't as easy as it should have been. I was technically a third-grader going into fourth grade. However, I only had one year in a traditional school, which was kindergarten. The school had supplied the tutor during first grade. She followed the curriculum set by the school. By all accounts, I was on track at the end of first grade. The school knew that. What was of concern was how much BOCES diverted from an average second- and third-grade curriculum.

How behind had I fallen? No one really knew. I'm not sure they wanted to know because they made no effort to find out. They heard I was in a wheelchair, frequently missed school and spent two years in a *special* school and went with their first assumption: I was irredeemably behind and couldn't catch up.

They gave mom two choices. First, they offered to have me repeat the third grade. That didn't sit well with her. She didn't want me to get left back when she had no indication that I needed to repeat the third grade. I hadn't failed. She was never told I was under-performing, even though in BOCES, grades were practically non-existent. The other option was putting me in special education classes. They said it would be for a short time to help me acclimate to the rigors of elementary school and catch up. What they didn't tell her was that in the late '80s, special education wasn't just a class, it was a label, and one I wouldn't free myself from until college. I know she thought she was choosing the lesser of the evils when she agreed to have me start fourth grade in special education.

Once I left BOCES, I couldn't have physical therapy in school three days a week. I did have it when all the other kids went to gym class. To supplement the therapy I was missing, my parents hired a physical therapist, Gracie. She would come to our home after school three days a week and give me physical therapy. Gracie specialized in pediatric physical therapy. I had more fun with her than I did with the rigid older physical therapist at BOCES. Her focus was less on me walking and more on building muscle strength, so much of which I lost during fracture healing and surgery.

The school assigned me an aid, Mrs. C, to help me in and around the school. She'd help me get things out of my backpack, which hung off the back of my wheelchair and was impossible for me to reach. If I had to go to the bathroom, she'd take me to the only accessible bathroom in the school and help me transfer on and off the toilet. She was super nice and very helpful, but she was an adult who followed me around. I hated that. Kids outside of the Special Ed class avoided me like the plague because Mrs. C was always just a few feet away. They thought she was watching them and would report any minor infraction to the principal. To the best of my knowledge, Mrs. C never acted as a spy, and she didn't have some covert operation to catch kids misbehaving. Regardless, nine-year-old girls aren't inclined to debate who is the cuter of the five New Kids on The Block with a 60-year-old woman, so I didn't have a lot of friends. I didn't leave the Special Ed classroom. In place of gym, I got physical therapy. I was exempt from gym because the last thing you want the little girl with Brittle Bone Disease doing is playing dodge ball.

I almost didn't care that I didn't make many friends. I was social, but I gravitated towards adults. I was constantly surrounded by adults: doctors, nurses, and X-ray techs were a huge part of my childhood. I spent more time in the hospital than I did at sleepovers. So there was an ease I had around adults. I spent most of my free time chatting up Mrs. C and the teachers. They'd listen dutifully as I told them about my life, my little sister, our dog and the latest episode of *Mr. Wizard* I'd watched. I loved science, so I loved that show.

***

Mom would tell the story of the day I made a "volcano" in a cup for years. One Saturday morning, Ashley and I had woken up before everyone else. I asked her if she wanted to do an experiment. I had seen Mr. Wizard make a "volcano." I crawled into the kitchen and persuaded Ashley to climb on one of the kitchen chairs and hand me the baking soda, vinegar and a cup. Sure, Mr. Wizard had a plaster volcano model, but I had to work with what I had. I filled the cup with vinegar and haphazardly just poured in the baking soda. I was thrilled when I saw the chemical reaction as the mixture started to fizz and bubble. It started to spill over and out of the cup. I was now sitting in a puddle of my vinegar and baking soda concoction. For reasons I'll never understand, Ashley burst into tears. She probably anticipated that mom would be pissed. Mom didn't like unnecessary messes. Mom heard all the commotion and woke up. When she got to the kitchen door, she stared, confused as to what she was actually looking at. I was sitting in a huge puddle. I think she thought I peed on myself.

"It's a chemical reaction, mom!" I proclaimed. "This is what happens when you mix an acid and a base," I said, clearly proud of my scientific accomplishment.

"This is a mess," she replied, scooping me up to go change my clothes.

She hated the mess, but she appreciated my ingenuity. I couldn't get off the floor, so I was able to enlist my sister to get me the supplies I needed to make a mess.

***

At school, the teachers never got to see that ingenuity. They never even asked me questions. It felt as if they didn't expect I'd be able to answer. I wanted to tell them that I wanted to be an astronaut. I hoped to be the first human to land on Mars.

I'd learn this is a common complaint among disabled people. Almost all will tell you that they were rarely asked what they wanted to be when they grew up, as if we were going to stay disabled children forever.

I got sick of waiting for people to engage me and became really good at engaging others and telling them what I wanted them to know. There was so much more to me than broken bones, surgeries and a wheelchair. I wanted people to know that. I was beginning to understand that I was in a box, and adults could only see the disabled child I was. They didn't' have the frame of reference that would allow them to envision me becoming a fully functioning, independent woman.

***

I had one friend my age, Lorna. I met Lorna at BOCES. She was the best thing to come out of my time there. Lorna was a wheelchair user like me. She was smart as a whip and probably one of the funniest people I ever met. We would have sleepovers during the weekends and just laugh. Her father would take us out. He'd take us to the movies or lunch.

He never seemed to mind being our go-to chaperone. He just let us be friends. Not disabled friends. Just friends. He was brave enough to venture into NYC with two prepubescent disabled girls giggling the whole time. Lorna was proof to me that I wasn't an oddity. You could not be able to walk and still be intelligent.

***

By fifth grade, things were marginally better for me. I was still in Special Ed, but things were changing. I was trying to assert some independence. Mrs. C felt it was her job to always push my wheelchair. I hated that. It made me feel like a baby in a stroller. Other kids thought they could push me too. They'd sneak up behind me and start pushing me. It felt like I was being kidnapped. Nobody would walk up to a child walking and just pick them up and start walking away. I demanded mom take the handlebars off of my wheelchair. She never pushed me anyway. When I was out with my family, I pushed myself. I never got tired or asked for help. Mom knew that and removed them.

***

When Mrs. C retired, the school replaced her with a new aide, Betty Yorie. Betty was much younger, about my parents' age. She gave me a lot more autonomy. She would only help me with something that I asked for help with. Even when I thought I could do more than I could, Betty waited for me to concede and ask for help. I was also blessed to end up in Barbara Lazzaro's class. Mrs. Lazzaro was like no other teacher I had before. She was the first teacher to believe in me. Mrs. Lazzaro knew she was teaching Special Ed, but that didn't stop her from seeing the potential in not just me, but all her students. She was the first adult outside of my family to ask me what I wanted to be when I grew up. When I told her I wanted to be an astronaut, she didn't rattle off all the reasons I wouldn't be able to do that. Instead, she replied,"You can! You'll have to get good grades in school so you can go to a good college. So work hard."

She was the first person to say the word "college" to me. That's also the first time someone equated how much effort I put into school to how much academic success I could have. Prior to that, everyone had acted like my academic success was predetermined by my disability.

You Just Do What Needs To Be Done

If my story has a hero, it's my mom. Deborah A. Faulk is one of the most selfless women to walk the face of this earth. Stories floated around the family about how she always fed stray dogs and invited kids who had less than her family to dinner at her house nightly. My uncle called her a "bleeding heart." My mom hated the inequities in this world. She proudly spoke of attending marches and rallies organized by members of the Black Panther Party. She would give you the shirt off her back—but don't cross her or her family. If you did, she'd raise hell. Living through the Civil Rights era, and loathing the inequities that she experienced, positioned her to be my biggest ally and fiercest advocate.

In fifth grade, I had the opportunity to join the school band. I wanted to play the clarinet because that's what my cousin Brandie played. Brandie was eight years older than me and the epitome of '80s cool. I wanted to be just like her. If she liked it, I loved it. The clarinet wouldn't work because of the foot rest on my wheelchair. So I decided I'd try the flute. I met with the band teacher, who immediately said, "I don't think you'll be able to hold the flute."

My arms are bowed and I have limited mobility in both wrists. It made sense that she would say that. Undeterred, I wanted to try anyway. She placed the flute in my hands and instructed me to hold it out to the left. I tried, but my arms just couldn't rotate enough to hold it like that.

"Yeah, band won't work for you," the band teacher said.

I was so deflated. Tears immediately welled up in my eyes. I left the band room feeling defeated and angry. I cried the whole way home.

When I got home, Gracie was there. I just learned I couldn't be in the school band *and* it was therapy day?

I didn't want to work on leg strength or balance, which was a typical session. I asked Gracie if she could help me with my arms. She was confused. She told me there was nothing wrong with my arm strength. I push a manual wheelchair every day, I explained. I needed help "turning them over" so I could hold the flute. She told me I should have no problem holding the flute.

"But I do," I said, as I tried to position my arms to hold an imaginary flute out to the left.

"Is that how they told you to hold it?" Gracie asked.

I nodded, still feeling defeated. Gracie explained that is not how you hold the flute. The flute is held out to the right. Gracie's daughter played the flute in her school band so she was certain. She gently positioned my arms to the right, holding my imaginary flute. I stayed frozen like that for a moment. I couldn't understand why a teacher would tell me to hold the flute backward. *Was it an innocent mistake?* She taught music for a living, but everybody had off days. *Did she not like me?* I zoned out thinking of every possible scenario for why a teacher would set me up for failure.

Gracie broke my daze when she uttered the words that would set mom off: "She didn't want to teach you!"

I got a knot in the pit of my stomach. I felt awful. Why would a teacher not want to teach *me?*

"This is discrimination! This will not stand!" Mom shouted.

The Americans With Disabilities Act (ADA) was a few months away from being signed. However, President Ford signed IDEA (Individuals With Disabilities Education Act) into law in 1975. That law guaranteed me an equal education. Gracie explained that, under the law, if all fifth graders were allowed to play an instrument, the school is legally obligated to teach me to play an instrument too. That was all mom needed to hear. Armed with that information, she put me on the bus the next day with plans of her own.

Uninvited and without an appointment, mom showed up at the school demanding to speak with the Principal. Mr. Quinn was an older docile man at the end of his career, and he was doing all he could to keep that school together. He was no match for a sharp-tongued black woman who could breathe fire to defend her family. He took the impromptu meeting with her anyway. She gave Mr. Quinn a crash course in IDEA. She threatened every possible legal action if I was not given an equal opportunity to play an instrument.

"I will make so much noise that your great grandchildren, who aren't even born yet, will know you stood for discrimination!" She told him.

Before that week was over, the band teacher asked me to join her in the band room. I was nervous about that. I knew mom had spoken to Mr. Quinn about what happened.

Did the teacher get in trouble? Did she want to confront me about it?

I really wanted to learn how to play the flute, so I hoped that she was going to invite me to join the band. That's exactly what she did. Without making any mention of the first time I was in this room when she told me to hold the flute backward, she told me I could take band. I wanted to be happy about that, but I struggled. I couldn't get past the fact that I knew she didn't want me in band originally. It wasn't as if there were band auditions and I just wasn't good enough to get in. She hadn't even let me try. I knew the only reason I was going to be in band was that she most likely faced repercussions.

It wasn't just band. Mom went to Mr. Quinn for the slightest infraction. Once, the toilet in the accessible bathroom wasn't working, so I had to use the bathroom in the nurse's office. I told mom about that, and like clockwork, she showed up at Mr. Quinn's office the next day. I swear she had that man's number on speed dial, but still preferred to confront him face to face.

Mr. Quinn announced his retirement in the middle of fifth grade. As a family, we joked about it. I was in my last year of elementary school. Mr. Quinn just had to make it until June, and he'd be done with this disabled student and her mother. However, Ashley would start Kindergarten in the same school. Dad said he retired because he was unwilling to deal with "Deborah Faulk: The Sequel." I doubt that's true, but mom certainly did not make his last year at that school pleasant.

***

Mr. Quinn was not the only person who drew mom's ire. She waged war with insurance companies on a daily basis. High insurance deductibles, denied treatments and uncovered durable medical equipment threatened to bankrupt my parents before I reached high school. It was clear the HMO my dad had through his job wasn't sufficient. It seemed like mom was on the phone fighting an insurance denial every day, checking the status of preauthorization for my physical therapy or begging for payment plans from doctors I had seen whose visits weren't covered for one reason or another.

***

With Ashley about to start school, and me already being in school full-time, mom could return to the workforce. Mom had a degree from the Fashion Institute of Technology in fashion design. That came in super handy because due to my tiny size, she couldn't find clothes in the store that fit me. Mom designed and made all of my clothes. She had a dream of being a fashion designer. She wanted a runway show during New York City's Fashion Week. I have no doubt that she could have done it. She was incredibly talented. She almost never needed a pattern. She would dream up an outfit for me, draw it on paper and cut her own patterns out of newspapers. After a few hours behind the sewing machine, she would have a finished product. It was borderline amazing watching her sew.

Every time inspiration struck, I got a new outfit. My favorite was a powder blue skirt with a matching sweater that resembled a cheerleader's uniform. I'd wear that with lace cutoff tights and felt like I was at the height of '80s fashion. Unfortunately for her, life got in the way. She was married with her first baby all before her twenty-fourth birthday. She'd received my life-changing diagnosis before she even turned thirty. She had no time for dreams. She had to be practical.

She looked for jobs that offered the best benefits, mainly health care. She quickly learned that the most comprehensive benefits packages and top-tier health insurance came from civil service jobs. I don't know how she found it, but mom took a job with the Suffolk County Police Department as a corrections officer. She worked out of a local precinct. As part of her job, she strip-searched and watched newly arrested women. She worked the 11 p.m. to 7 a.m. shift.

Every night after dinner, my petite five-foot six-inch mother would get dressed in her uniform: black pants and a white shirt with a gold and black "Suffolk County PD" patch affixed just below both shoulders. She'd pin on her badge and put on the thick black belt that completed her uniform. On the left side, that belt held her handcuffs, and on the right, it held her nightstick. Her tiny frame was swallowed up by that uniform. The contrast between the feminine, warm and gentle woman I knew and the no-nonsense, tough-as-nails corrections officer she'd become at night was stark. It was like watching Bruce Wayne turn into Batman. She'd get Ashley and me ready for school and put us on the bus. Then, she would sleep until we got home. She'd wake up, help with homework, cook dinner and do it all over again.

That job took a toll on her mentally and emotionally. She dealt with girls, often only a few years older than her own daughters, who'd been arrested for drug offenses or prostitution. She met girls who were 16 and 17 and had to search them to make sure they weren't hiding drugs in their vaginas. She hated that. She would say that she often felt like many of those girls were victims and she was asked to strip them of the last bit of dignity they had left.

One morning, she bought home a tiny origami swan. I asked where she'd gotten it. She told me that a 16-year-old girl had been arrested the night before for buying heroin. She had called her parents to come bail her out. They refused. She was in the holding cell crying. Being a mother herself, I think her maternal instinct just took over. She talked to this girl most of the night. The girl asked if she could have some paper. My mom gave her a piece of paper from a tiny pad she had. The girl then carefully crafted that little paper swan and gave it to my mom before her shift was over the next morning. That origami swan sat on my mom's dresser for years.

I think my mom believed she was making a difference. Even if none of those girls remembered her, she hoped she was having some impact. Before going home, she would tell every girl on her watch, "I better not see you here again."

She hated that job. Every night, she'd groan and mutter to herself about how she didn't want to go. If anything got her through those nights, it was the lofty idea that somehow interacting with these girls, humanizing them and listening to their stories would somehow be the catalyst to turn their lives around.

One night while she was getting ready for work, I heard her complaining to herself about being tired and not wanting to go. I was a kid and couldn't comprehend why anyone would do something they loathed so much. Mom was clearly miserable, and the exhaustion was visible.

"Mom, if you hate this job so much, why do you go?" I asked her.

She looked me square in the eye and said, "Taniya, you're not going to like everything in life. But sometimes you just do what needs to be done."

I love her for that mindset, but I'd be lying if I said I didn't feel guilty that she sacrificed so much. She put her children above all else. Even when that meant she was last on her own list of priorities.

The new job did mean additional income and great health insurance. We finally got out of our cramped two-bedroom apartment. My grandfather purchased a five-bedroom, two-story home and rented it out to my parents. I also got a brand new wheelchair that was custom-fit for me. Although I only had it for two years, I had already grown out of my first wheelchair. Because the new one was custom-fit, it had to be ordered so I got to pick the color. A neon pink frame with black wheels. You would have thought I was getting my first car. That's how excited I was to pick it up.

The new house was great. Ashley and I got our own bedrooms, plus a separate playroom. It had a huge backyard with plenty of space for a swing set and pool. We even got a dog, an oversized German Shepard that mom named Chardonnay. Mom named a huge mean-looking dog after a delicate white wine and we just all went along with it. We called her "Chardy." Chardonnay was just way too much to say every time you called a dog. She was a great dog. Supper sappy and sweet, even though she looked like one of those vicious police dogs on TV. She was very protective of us. Ashley and I tried to teach her how to pull my wheelchair until mom reminded me: *she's a guard dog, not a sled dog!*

We looked like everything you thought American families should look like: two kids, a dog and a white picket fence. There was just one problem: none of it was accessible. There were steps outside leading to the front door. Once inside, there were two flights of stairs—ones that went up to the main portion of the house and ones that went down to the den and the playroom. My wheelchair couldn't fit through any of the doorways. It was as if everybody involved in choosing and agreeing to move in this house unintentionally forgot that a disabled kid was going to live there.

If the endgame was to ensure that I became as independent as possible, this house was the perfect tool to facilitate that. I know that sounds extremely counter-intuitive: *how could a house that I couldn't freely move around allow my independence to blossom?* I couldn't even get into my own bedroom or down the stairs without help. The answer: sometimes you just do what needs to be done!

I knew that if I wanted to get somewhere, I was going to have to figure it out. I learned to just abandon my wheelchair in the foyer, like a pair of dirty shoes that you don't wear in the house. I'd slide down from the seat to the footrest and then the floor. I'd bear-crawl up the stairs. I stayed on the floor, crawling everywhere I needed to go. I don't know if she sensed how liberating that was or if she was self-disciplined enough to know not to blur the line between helping and hindering, but mom just let me be. She basically refused to carry me around. She trusted me to figure it out, and that made all the difference.

There were only two scenarios in which she would pick me up: getting on the toilet and getting in bed. Our bathrooms had beautiful beige ceramic tile floors. There is no doubt that if I fell in there, I'd sustain multiple fractures. Even though Ashley and I had our own rooms, we still wanted to sleep together. Mom got us bunk beds. Almost immediately I claimed the top bunk. Maybe it was childhood optimism. I couldn't even walk, certainly I wasn't going to climb a ladder. I just knew I was the oldest so I had dibs on the top bunk. In typical mom fashion, she wasn't going to stop me from doing something. Every night, she'd pick me up and put me in bed and every morning she'd come get me out. I'd dread the nights when I'd wake up having to use the bathroom. I'd have to lie there yelling for mom and dad to come get me and take me. They were both hard sleepers, so sometimes even my best efforts were futile. Luckily, Ashley was just a few feet beneath me. I'd drop something between the wall and my bed and it would land on her bed. She'd be startled awake by the dirty tissue, Barbie or sock that seemingly fell from nowhere. Once she was up, I'd ask her to go get mom or dad, and she would.

***

Ashley contributed to my independence when we were children in ways she never understood. I couldn't play in our backyard in my wheelchair. The terrain wasn't level, and we had a mole problem so every few feet, one of the front casters on my chair would sink into a mole hole and my chair would tip forward. But we also had this old-school Radio Flyer wagon. I'd get in it, and she'd pull me anywhere we wanted to play. She was always super nice to me and dutifully pulled me around. However, she also used that wagon to take out her grievances on me. Once, she was mad at me about something so she pulled me all the way down our 70-foot driveway to the patch of grass behind our mailbox. She left me there and ran to the house.

Even though she was five years younger than me, she was bigger than me. Not only was she taller, but she was an overweight kid. Something about us together gave my mom comfort. When we were together, she didn't worry nearly as much as if we were on our own. Ashley couldn't fight her way out of a paper bag, but mom viewed her as my protector. One time, she broke a stick over the back of a neighborhood boy who was making fun of me. Ashley would hop on her bike and ride along with me in my chair and we'd ride to the nearest 7-11 for Slurpees in the summer. All the kids on our block had bikes. I had my wheelchair. I knew it wasn't the same, but it felt equal. I'd offer to race any kid on a bike any day. They all let me, thinking there was no way a set of arms pushing a manual wheelchair could beat them. More often than not, I came out victorious.

***

That house offered what I never knew I was missing: a sense of normalcy and independence. Our previous apartment was so small that I had no need to really move around. It was easy to pick me up and carry me from the couch into the kitchen and from the kitchen into the bedroom. It was all only separated by a few feet. In this house, I wanted to move freely and explore. I finally had friends who were my age. There was a sense of normalcy in that I almost forgot to feel abnormal.

When strangers stared at me, or an inquisitive child asked, "Why can't you walk?" that's when the illusion of normalcy would fall away. I remained unfazed by most of the stares. I reconciled it by telling myself that I still found it hard not to stare at people who used wheelchairs. I'd stare out of the sheer wonder of seeing someone who moved like me. It was the "Why can't you walk?" line of questioning that bothered me.

Because that was a question with an answer I didn't have. I wasn't always in a wheelchair, and I wasn't old enough that I had forgotten the time I spent walking. I had vivid memories of playing Hop Scotch with Julie, running and skating. Over the course of those first years as a wheelchair user, I mourned that loss. At the time, I couldn't verbalize it, but I felt robbed of something. I knew something was *taken* from me and I didn't know why.

When kids asked, "Hey, why can't you walk?" what I wanted to say was, "I really don't know! Something went wrong, I guess?" Instead, I replied,"Because I have Osteogenesis Imperfecta. God made me this way."

That was a perfect, kid-friendly answer to a painfully awkward question. Except I didn't believe that. God hadn't made me a kid who couldn't walk. God took a kid who could walk and run and turned her into a kid who couldn't walk. I knew the *how* was because God gave me Osteogenesis Imperfecta. I didn't understand the *why.*

Baby Steps

My parents were one hundred percent committed to my physical therapy regimen from the start. Even when I wavered on wanting to go, they were all in. The problem was they didn't feel the exhaustion and soreness that followed every session. They would bring me ice packs and Tylenol. So they knew it was painful, but they didn't *feel* it. I got physical therapy in school in place of gym on Tuesdays and Thursdays. Gracie came to my house after school on Mondays, Wednesdays and Fridays, and I received aqua therapy at an outpatient facility on Saturdays, as long as I wasn't in a cast. Physical therapy is hard, grueling work. Often, I was rehabbing a freshly healed fracture. After six or eight weeks in a cast, the muscle in the area atrophies. Almost every time I healed from a fracture, the muscle atrophy would be so intense that it would render the limb practically useless. I'd set off on the daunting task of making the limb functional again.

Not every session was aimed at rehabilitating an injury. Most weren't. Physical therapy offered my parents something they had very little of: control. They couldn't control if or when I fractured a bone. But they could control what they did to help. By having me in physical therapy as often as possible, and exposing me to various therapeutic modalities, my parents had an active role in my healing, or at least I felt like they did.

My parents were also fed that late '80s narrative about life for disabled adults being borderline impossible to live independently and be successful. We were navigating the perils of life as a family with a disabled American in the years prior to the Americans with Disabilities Act being signed. We couldn't foresee the life an adult me could have, when everything in the life of 10-year-old me was inconvenient. Access was virtually impossible at some places.

We took a field trip to historic Philadelphia. The school required mom to come as my chaperone, or I couldn't go. Without saying as much, they were unwilling to take the liability of taking me off school property and out of state for a day. I know she didn't want to, but as always, she did what needed to be done to allow me to have a normal childhood experience. All of the typical tourist attractions were on the day's agenda: The Liberty Bell, Independence Hall and The Betsy Ross

House. I was immediately struck by the old sidewalks and cobblestone streets. My wheelchair kept getting stuck in the cracks in the concrete. I felt so uneasy, as if at any moment my chair was going to tip over.

When we got to Betsy Ross's House, I was greeted by a flight of stairs leading to the entranceway. That feeling I felt when I couldn't navigate my way around was unmatched. It almost felt like the world was telling me, *you're not wanted here.* I could understand that the world just wasn't built for me, but at times, it was like the world was built *intentionally* against me.

Undeterred, mom looked at me and said, "Don't worry, leave it there."

I looked around, baffled. Surely she didn't mean I should just abandon this $3,000 wheelchair that she had to fight the insurance company to cover. *Did she really mean we were just going to leave it on the front lawn of the Betsy Ross House?*

That's exactly what she meant! She walked over to me, picked me up in her arms, and carried me inside the house. She effortlessly walked in and out of the rooms while holding me. She carefully navigated the narrow staircase up to the bedrooms. I could feel her breath quicken. I couldn't tell if she was nervous that she'd trip or if she was exerting more energy trying to comfortably hold me and walk up a flight of stairs. Regardless, I knew she was struggling. I began to feel guilty and wanted to tell her to just put me down. But this wasn't my house with its plush carpeting and open floor plan. I wouldn't be able to safely crawl around this space.

That is the moment I connected my ability to walk to my independence. I saw the two as intricately connected and mutually exclusive.

***

I wanted to walk. I told everyone who'd listen that I would walk again. I didn't *really* want to walk. I wanted all the things I thought walking would give me. I wanted to take dance classes like Ashley. I wanted to run with Julie. I wanted to actually be able to hide during hide and seek. You can't exactly hide behind a tree in a neon pink wheelchair. I wanted to be independent. Most importantly though I was consumed with not letting all the doctors who said I couldn't, wouldn't, or shouldn't walk be right. Even then, the quickest way to get me to do something was to tell me I couldn't do it. I was competitive by nature. Just the idea of defeat was enough motivation to push me for months. When Mom or Gracie asked me, "Do you want to walk?" What I heard was, "Do you want the doctors who said you'd never walk, the ones who said you would die, the music teacher who didn't want you in band, the people who recommended *special* schools to be right about you?"

Once I internalized that thought, walking became a priority. I threw myself into my physical therapy. Gracie found herself met with very little resistance. Countless sessions began with me sitting on a medicine ball as Gracie held her arms outstretched, ready to catch me if I fell.

"Sit up straight," she'd say. "Stabilize that core."

I had terrible balance. You don't really need balance when you roll around on four wheels all day. Gracie knew that if I was ever going to stand, I'd need to master balance first. It was a delicate and daunting task. Thank God Gracie had cat-like reflexes because she never let me hit the floor. If I tilted too far one way or the other, she'd gently grab me. That was some magical power she had. She could touch me with strength and not cause me to fracture. At that time, that was no easy feat. Maybe it was her education. After all, she was a licensed physical therapist. She should know how to not injure patients. I wasn't an average patient, though, and very little was known about OI and how to handle patients with it. When she would manually stretch my legs to release some of the tension in my hamstrings, I'd calmly surrender.

Gracie was safe. I knew she was safe, and I trusted her. Gracie was also naturally maternal and really cared. My learning to walk mattered to her as much as it did to my parents.

After years of that medicine ball, combined with leg lifts and stretching, Gracie got me on my feet. She had me transfer out of my wheelchair to a small ottoman we had in the living room. The only time my wheelchair ever made it past the foyer of my house was when I was practicing transfers with Gracie. She placed one hand on each side of my waist and asked me to stand. I was absolutely terrified. It had been more than five years since I last felt the ground beneath my feet. I had broken so many bones just by standing. I knew the rods were supposed to prevent fractures, but I didn't trust them entirely. *How do you trust something you can't see?* The rods were more conceptual for me than anything. I couldn't see, touch or feel them in my bones, and I was being asked to trust that the rods would protect me. That was a big ask for a 10-year-old. Mom, who was standing in the corner of the room, looked at me with wild anticipation of what she was about to witness. She whispered, "Trust yourself. You can do this."

I inhaled deeply, filling my lungs with air as if the minute I stood up, I'd forget to breathe. I stood up and immediately looked down at my legs. Gracie still had her hands on my waist but wasn't holding that tightly. I couldn't believe my legs were holding me.

"Hey! Look up. When we walk, we have to look where we're going," Gracie said, when she saw me staring at my feet. She took her hands off my waist and held them up in front of me. "You're standing on your own. I'm not holding you!"

For the first time in six years, I could feel the weight of my own body. I wasn't weightless like I was in the pool during aqua therapy. I felt the heaviness of gravity. I felt what carpet feels like beneath your feet. I also felt what fatigue feels like. I only stood for about a minute, but I felt my quadriceps start to quiver and calf muscles begin to cramp. I don't know if it was because she saw me grit my teeth and wince, but Gracie placed her hands on my sides and told me to sit down. I collapsed with a sigh of relief on top of that ottoman.

As I sat there, I swelled with pride. I just did something that was deemed impossible. I'd won. In reality, I may have won the first battle in what would be a 30-year war. In the blink of an eye, Gracie had a pediatric walker at my house. I knew everything I got had to be approved by the insurance company well in advance. It was clear that this walker had to be in the works for weeks, if not months, prior to me standing. Gracie must have really believed in me, and the possibility that I would eventually walk.

Even my uncle, who only a few years earlier suggested I should be put in an institution, rallied behind me. I had a support system like never before. People were rooting for my success. I wasn't accustomed to that. I was used to the anticipation of failure before I even tried. The attention felt good. For the first time in my life, I felt people look at me with hope and optimism instead of pity. The only person who never pitied me was mom. People were finally starting to see me through her eyes. She saw possibilities when everyone else could only see problems for me.

I fed off the adulation and praise. The more people told me how proud they were, the more I wanted to do. I knew if simply standing could earn me so much positive attention, walking would surely be ten times better.

Those first few steps were fueled by ableism and the insatiable need I had for people to be proud of me. Everybody wanted me to get better. Let's face it though, there was no cure for Osteogenesis Imperfecta, and we all knew it. What they meant by wanting me to get better was that they wanted me to be *normal.* I don't fault my parents for that. Their subliminal ableist messaging was a byproduct of the time. In the '80s and '90s, disability and independence didn't coexist. How could I hold them accountable for not recognizing what the world could be but only seeing what it was? I wish they had noticed that everything I did was for validation. If I wasn't going to be praised for it, it almost didn't feel worth doing.

***

I barely used the walker in the house. I was supposed to practice, but that got old really fast. The wheels got stuck on the carpet, I just wasn't as fast as when I crawled, and I couldn't take it down the stairs. Getting around my house was just easier on the floor. When I was honest with myself, I didn't want to walk as much as I wanted people to see me walk.

At the time, I'm pretty sure mom, dad and Gracie all knew that. That's why it came as no surprise when I announced that I wanted to walk at the end of fifth grade for the moving up ceremony. All three of them nodded in agreement.

"You can do anything you set your mind to, girl!" Dad proclaimed.

Mom gave me her big toothy smile that she only gave when she was really happy or deeply approved of the topic being discussed. What they didn't realize was that the only reason I wanted to walk across the stage at the moving up ceremony was so I'd have an audience. It was not uncommon for people to stare at me. I was learning that I may not be able to control *when* strangers stared, but I could control the *why.*

***

On the day of the ceremony, the gym was packed with the families of all the fifth graders. I was parked in my wheelchair off to the side about 20 or 30 feet from the podium. I was on full display as every kid crossed to accept their certificate. As the principal started calling the "E's," I knew my name would be coming up soon. I undid my seatbelt, kicked up my footrest and slid to the edge of my wheelchair. With Gracie's assistance, I got to my feet and positioned myself in that walker. Then I heard my name.

"Taniya Faulk," the principal called.

I steadied myself and began to take tiny steps. I shuffled my feet one at a time like a toddler. When I got to the podium, I lifted one hand and accepted my certificate. The crowd erupted in applause and leaped to their feet. Even the other fifth graders were giving me a standing ovation. I basked in the moment, beaming with pride. I didn't know it then, but I had just fed a narrative that I would grow to loathe as an adult: adoring and praising disabled people for doing seemingly normal activities.

In reality, I know there was nothing normal about walking that day. By all early accounts, I wasn't even supposed to live to see my tenth birthday, never mind graduating fifth grade, and being on the cusp of my 11th birthday. I enjoyed the adulation, but I'm not sure I deserved it. Most of those people in that room didn't know me. They just knew they saw a handicapped girl walk, and certainly that was amazing. We were still in the day of Jerry Lewis and his Muscular Dystrophy telethons. I wasn't one of *Jerry's kids*. I didn't even share the same disability as the kids featured during those telethons. However, for the parents in that gym, I was about as close as they were going to get to a feel-good story or reason to appreciate their own *normal* kids a little more.

I knew for my family that moment was monumental. I'd defied all the odds: I was alive and I was walking. In five years, I'd come a long way. That couldn't be understated. What also could not be understated is how much further I would have to go. I naively thought this was the end. I'd break a few bones, get around with a walker and effortlessly move into adulthood and carve out a life for myself.

The road that lay ahead was about to be bumpier than anything I could imagine. God wrote a story and cast me in the starring role. I just didn't know the plot, but I'd quickly learn I would get to determine if this story was going to be a comedy or a tragedy.

House Of Cards

My parents' marriage was barely hanging on by a thread. They fought all the time. Theirs was a volatile relationship. At times, it was downright toxic.

Dad was an alcoholic who was often out of work. Money was always tight. At the heart of all their arguments was the reality that there were always more bills than there was money to pay them. Maybe it was because he was tired of the arguments or mom's nagging, or maybe he was annoyed that our cable was the first utility mom would cut off, but he would grab a newspaper and look for work. Dad would get a new job and they could breathe again. However, he'd be unemployed again and the cycle would start all over.

He wasn't exactly the most motivated individual. Every time he lost a job, he treated it like a well-earned vacation. He slept late, watched TV all day and just got lost in his favorite TV shows. Looking back, I see it was probably easier for him to lose himself in the worlds of The Andy Griffith Show and Bonanza. These were worlds without disabled kids, mounting medical debt and mundane daily life. He lived in the house, but I still felt very detached from him. I felt like the only time I could have him be present for me was when I was making physical gains towards *normal.* In hindsight, I don't think he wanted me to be *normal.* He wanted me to be *easier.* Easier to handle, easier to take places, easier to hug, easier to afford.

We all knew Dad drank too much, but we didn't talk about it. It was the family secret that we never questioned. Mom was the product of an alcoholic mother. To her, hiding family alcoholism was natural and normal. She fell into the unhealthy pattern of enabling his alcoholism. She was always done with him, but never *finished.* They perpetually split up and got back together more than high schoolers experiencing their first relationship. Ashley and I were constantly caught in the push and pull of it all. I always felt like I had to pick a side.

Siding with mom came naturally. During all those late-night runs to the emergency room and hospital stays when she never left my side, we bonded. In my eyes, she was a Goddess. She was strong, powerful and loved me beyond belief. Dad, on the other hand, held back out of fear. Fear of hurting me, fear of losing me and the overall fear of not knowing what happens next. I internalized what I perceived to be distance as a lack of love for me. I often asked mom if he loved me, to which she would always reply, "Of course." But she never attempted to explain his behavior to me. Maybe she didn't even understand it herself.

The distance between dad and I had grown bigger and deeper than ever. We barely spoke, and he had stopped going to doctor's appointments with us. He'd offer to stay at the house and watch Ashley, who was still young enough that she wasn't good at sitting still in office waiting rooms. It sounded like a viable reason, but in actuality, it was an excuse. Ashley offered Dad an escape that nobody knew he was looking for. He didn't have to look at X-rays, talk about broken bones or see me in pain. As a kid, that resonated as a lack of love for me. As an adult, I realize it's more likely that his love for me kept him away. Most often, when I was visiting a doctor, I was already in pain or about to experience pain. You have to be an incredibly strong person to watch helplessly as your child screams and cries in pain. Sometimes, Dad would push past his fears and come. He'd leave Ashley with his sister, our Aunt D, and Nana. As I got older, it became easier for him to be there. Ashley spent a lot of time with our Grandma too. In the same ways I felt like I only had mom, Ashley felt like she only had dad. We felt evenly divided.

***

Mom and Dad were polar opposites in how they handled what certainly was an unknown future. Dad just took a wait-and-see approach. He figured there'd be nothing he could do anyway. Mom was not nearly as laid back. She didn't believe that things were unknown, just *undone.* She didn't believe you waited for the future to just happen. You create the future. Even if it was just her need to feel in control, she truly was on a mission to create the future she wanted her children to have, and no disease was going to rob her of that. If that meant telling doctors how to do their jobs, scrutinizing every X-ray and working with a geneticist to build an extensive family tree in an attempt to identify where in the bloodline my OI came from, she did it.

They came up empty on where my OI came from. That didn't matter. Mom felt like she *did* something.

For years, mom operated as a single parent. We had two households: one in the hospital and the other in our home. She held them both together like a pro. She would become annoyed if she came home after another emergency and Dad hadn't picked up the toys Ashley and I didn't put away. I may have been disabled, but Ashley and I could make a real mess, and we weren't great at picking up behind ourselves.

If we came home from taking me to a doctor's appointment and Ashley still hadn't been fed lunch after Dad eagerly offered to stay with her, mom would be really annoyed. Mom always preferred leaving Ashley with Aunt D and Nana. They were planners, like her. They would never forget to feed Ashley lunch.

Mom was a mother with two young children, one of them severely disabled. She needed the extra body in the house. She needed an extra set of hands to lift me when she couldn't. She needed a second income. They stayed married because, logistically, it made sense. I don't think either of them was ever completely happy. I could tell by the way they always fought. I know it wasn't my fault, but my OI didn't give them much of a chance at being happy together. They were apart a lot. And when they were together, it wasn't easy as just leaving for a date night. While Ashley could easily stay with friends and family, it wasn't that easy for them to leave me with anyone. I always ran the risk of breaking something, and who else, besides my parents, would be okay with stabilizing a fracture, carrying me to the car and taking me to the emergency room? It took a long time before they'd leave me with a babysitter, and even then it was only out of absolute necessity. They didn't go out much.

***

During her time at the police department, my mom saw so many wayward girls get caught up in drugs and prostitution. She recognized that many of them shared a single common denominator: they didn't have families. They were often homeless and without any true guidance. I know she wanted to help. My mother would have tried to save the world if she could.

***

Mom and Dad had their problems, and at times, those problems seemed insurmountable. They were the happiest when we were doing family things. Whether we were splashing each other at the pool or just barbecuing in our backyard, they were happy. If it was fun and lighthearted, they could get along great. Dad was really silly. He was like one big six-foot-tall kid. For mom, that was a blessing and a curse. He knew how to make her laugh. He also knew how to drive her insane. When Dad went from being goofy and silly to irresponsible and lazy, she'd call him her third child. Maybe children bind you together because if not for Ashley and me, they would have divorced. She didn't think he was perfect. She didn't even think he was a great provider. She did think he was a good father. She understood his avoidance and fears when it came to me, and she never held that against him.

***

It wasn't a surprise when she looked around at the five bedrooms we had, three completely unused because Ashley and I would rather share, and she signed up to be an emergency foster parent. I wonder if at that time she was merely looking for a distraction. By all standards, I was doing better. It was possible for me to go a few months without a fracture, all planned, preventative surgeries had been completed, and while I'd been her full-time project for six years, she suddenly had more free time than she knew what to do with. She had a lot of love to give, and may have actually had more kids after Ashley if OI wasn't part of the equation.

We had a few foster kids stay with us for short periods of time. Mom made it a point to take in older kids because everybody wanted babies and she was well aware that the 12, 13 and 14-year-olds were just a few years younger than the girls she'd have to watch in a jail cell overnight. Child Protective Services would place a kid who was in dire straits with emergency foster parents until CPS could find them permanent placement. The whole nature of the foster care system is temporary. It was nice for me to have someone else to play with besides Ashley. These kids were closer to my age, but one day, we'd get the word that they had found a permanent home and would be leaving. We'd say a quick goodbye and then they would be gone forever. I'd try to keep in touch by writing letters, but never heard back. I doubt those letters ever made it to their intended recipients.

Suddenly, mom decided she'd go further. She wanted to adopt a child, a little boy. Dad always talked about how badly he wanted a son. Right after Ashley was born, mom had her tubes tied. She made no excuses, she was done having babies! I was breaking bones every few weeks at that point so her hands were full. When my official diagnosis came down, and they were told it was genetic, she was secure in that decision. As far as she was concerned, they dodged a bullet by Ashley not having OI. With no definitive genetic test for OI, they had no way of knowing how or why I got it. Either me having OI or Ashley not having it was a fluke. If they had another biological child, there was no telling if that child would or would not have it. Even if she could have had another child, I don't think she would have.

She found Idris, a 2-year-old little boy listed with an adoption agency in New York City. His picture and bio were listed in a book of children available for adoption in New York. He was born addicted to crack, and his birth mom was serving time in a state prison. He was in a foster home in the Bronx. His story is what drew mom to him. She'd heard similar stories before from women who were arrested and had delivered babies addicted to drugs. Within weeks, we were on a train headed to New York City to meet him. He was the sweetest little boy. I loved him instantly. I was already an older sister, but Ashley wasn't a baby anymore. She was more my playmate. He was still in diapers. He was a real baby. I envisioned all the things I would teach him. Mom and dad were already approved foster parents, and they'd passed all the home visits and social worker interviews so he was able to move in relatively fast. He fit in with our family like he'd been there forever. Mom adored him, but hated his given name. She was resigned that he was going to be her son so she went about compiling names like an expectant mother.

Tevon Campbell was my favorite singer. One day, as if I had any say, I asked, "What about Tevon, mom?" Much to my surprise, she liked it and immediately renamed him Tevon Pharaoh Faulk. And just like that, we were a family of five.

Mean Girls

I started middle school, still in special education. My aide Betty followed me to middle school. With all the nervousness that accompanies starting middle school, Betty was my one constant. I was so glad I got to keep her. She was terrific. Mom worked with her husband, who was a cop. Betty gave me freedom. She wasn't one of those *do-gooder* adults who forced help upon me. It also helped that most of the kids liked her. Regardless, I still knew I was the middle school kid with an adult trailing behind.

Mom had worried that as I got older, I'd be bullied. She anticipated that my wheelchair would be the cause of the teasing and that I wouldn't be able to handle it. She was right to fear I'd have to deal with bullies. All kids can possibly encounter bullies. What she completely misjudged was *why* I would be bullied. Most of the kids barely mentioned my wheelchair. What drew their attention was my race or what they perceived to not be my race.

Being a black girl, mom prepared me for racism and what white supremacy might look like. She taught me that the world wasn't always fair when it came to race. She told Ashley and I stories of her childhood; stories about being at her grandmother's house in Virginia and being called names. She was old enough to remember when schools were first integrated, and although "Separate but Equal" was no longer an upheld doctrine, it was still a mindset. When she was young, she participated in marches organized by local activists. I remember extensive conversations with my mom about race. I viewed her as an expert on the subject of race. What she never told me was that there was a possibility that I may not be *black enough* for some people.

Longwood Middle School was comprised of mostly black students, and it was a part of the school district I'd been in since Kindergarten. I never had any problems in elementary school. Maybe it's because little kids are nicer. Maybe it's because I spent most of my early years being tutored and then at BOCES. Regardless, 11 and 12-year-olds get mean and look for anything to pick on you about. The wheelchair was the low-hanging fruit. I'm not sure why they didn't go after me for that. Perhaps it was too easy, too obvious. Maybe they anticipated I'd be ready for those quips with a fully formed response crafted to shut them down.

Instead, they chose to attack my *blackness.*

"Why do you talk like that?" they'd ask.

"You sound like a white girl!" they'd shout every time I opened my mouth.

I didn't know what they meant by that.

How does one sound like any particular race?

I didn't use any slang if that's what they meant. I wasn't allowed to, or rather I had to be prepared for the consequences if I did. If I let mom hear me say the word "ain't," I'd be fully prepared to lose access to whatever television show she thought I got it from. Plus, Nana was a stickler for pronunciation and diction. If I mispronounced a word in front of her, she would say, "Excuse me, what?" And I'd have to repeat the entire sentence until I realized or corrected my mistake.

I was also continuously trying to prove my intelligence. The bigger a word was, the more often I'd use it. I was groomed to believe that proper English was expected whenever I opened my mouth, and big words were an indicator of high intelligence. Yet, here was this group of black girls who were insisting that those things were synonymous with being white. I couldn't reconcile the two.

In addition to sounding white, I guess, in their eyes, I didn't look black or black enough. Most of the women on dad's side of the family had long hair, especially the little girls. Dad made Ashley and I keep our hair long. He loved it. He loved to brush it and pet it. It was like some weird grooming ritual you'd see a cheetah do to a cub at the zoo. Mom always had medium to short haircuts. But dad had that archaic belief that a girl's femininity was tied to long, flowing locks. I wanted a haircut for years, but mom refused. She always relaxed our hair, straightened it with a hot comb and pulled it up into a high ponytail. In part, it was just easier for her to maintain. As long as it was relaxed, she'd take the hot comb to it on a Sunday and pull it up in a ponytail before we got on the bus every morning. I hated that ponytail! One day, one of the girls who called me a white girl daily decided she hated my ponytail too.

"I know her hair is fake," she announced to the class.

The teacher admonished her briefly before returning to the lesson. I had stopped thinking about it until I felt a tug on my ponytail. I whipped my head around as she withdrew her hand. She had just pulled my ponytail, expecting it to come off.

"It's really my hair!" I said sheepishly, not wanting to upset her.

Because of all of this, I was thrust into what I can only describe as an identity crisis. I didn't truly look like anyone I knew. I was so tiny, extremely thin, and relatively short for my age. There was also the hot pink wheelchair. I wasn't represented in any facets of pop culture. There were no singers, actors or anyone in the public arena who I could identify with. There weren't even very many toys or dolls that were designed to look like me. The closest I got to seeing myself reflected back at me was in the faces of the black girls I went to school with, and they hated me!

I tried to be smart, but I wasn't smart enough. I tried to walk, but I couldn't walk enough. The one thing I just was, the thing I thought I didn't have to try to be, was black. Suddenly, I realized that was wrong. No matter what I did, who I was or what I looked like by someone else's metric, I fell short. It was easy to tell myself that no one else's thoughts or opinions mattered. It was much harder to believe that. Like any other middle schooler, I just wanted to fit in. I probably would have been anything anybody wanted me to be if it meant I would be accepted. I didn't yet know that acceptance doesn't come from abandoning your authenticity, and shape-shifting into some watered-down version of yourself in an effort to be liked. That's exactly what I did. I was so sick of being told, "You're like an Oreo. Black on the outside, but white on the inside." I tried to act "blacker," but I didn't even know what that meant.

Was it a way of talking? Dressing? Thinking? Was blackness a behavior I could learn?

***

One day, I had to leave school early for a doctor's appointment. Mom, having worked all night, slept while me, Ashley and Tevon were at school. She sent dad to pick me up from school.

My father is a light-skinned black man. He was considerably lighter than my mom, which is what gave Ashley and I our medium-brown complexion. My dad had been mistaken for a person of Hispanic descent, but never white. That is until this particular day. One of the girls who tortured me daily saw him walking alongside me as I made my way to the front of the building. The bell had already rung, so the halls were relatively empty. That didn't stop her from trying to humiliate me.

"That's why you got that good hair. You got that white daddy!" she shouted.

I felt my cheeks get warm. I was embarrassed and I didn't know why.

Was I embarrassed by my father? Was I embarrassed that he didn't defend me? Why doesn't he just shout back, "I'm not white and neither is she!"

As an adult, I know that 40-year-old men shouldn't confront 12-year-old girls, but in that moment, I wanted to feel defended and protected. I wanted him to stand up for me! But he didn't. I knew if mom was there, she wouldn't have kept quiet. Mom was always armed with a snappy comeback for every occasion. Instead, dad just muttered, "Don't worry about it," as we walked out the oversized doors.

For the rest of middle school, that was the narrative that followed me: I had a white dad. For the kids that liked calling me white girl, this made sense. They'd doubted my blackness from the start, so seeing me with a much lighter-skinned man painted a picture that made them feel confident in their assertions.

I knew my dad wasn't white. I knew I wasn't biracial. The closest I was to being mixed was having Native American ancestry. That's not rare, though. What natural-born American doesn't have Native American blood running through their veins?

I internalized the attacks on my race. I barely spoke about it. How could I tell my mom, an unapologetic and proud black woman, that people thought her oldest daughter was white?

Would she be ashamed of me? Did I act like a white girl? Those thoughts echoed in my head often.

I thought it might be easier to just be white, and not for the reason one might think. Maybe it would just be easier to exist and just be who I was, speak how I spoke and not have my authenticity questioned if I were white.

Why couldn't I be closer to dad's complexion?

In a ridiculously futile effort to assimilate and feel like I belonged among the handful of white girls in the school, I studied the movie *Buffy the Vampire Slayer*. I watched it dozens of times. I mastered the stereotypical "Valley Girl" vernacular. I sounded like a ridiculous caricature of what I interpreted as whiteness. I changed my name twice. First, I wanted to be called Buffy. A few girls obliged and called me that but hearing it, I thought it made me sound dumb. So I changed my name for a second time to Brooke.

"I'm changing my name to Brooke! If you call me anything besides Brooke, I'm not answering!" I yelled from my bedroom

In retrospect, it was such a passive-aggressive 12-year-old move, but I thought I sounded serious and convincing. That was until mom called us for dinner.

"Ashley, Taniya, dinner in five!" She bellowed from the kitchen.

"My name's Brooke! I'm only answering to Brooke from now on!" I hollered back.

"Taniya LaSchaun Faulk, I am not calling you anything besides the name I gave you! Now get your butt in here so we can eat!" she replied sharply.

Like any mother, if she used my middle name, she meant business. I ate dinner with my family, abandoning my Brooke persona in my bedroom for the evening.

Later that night, mom confronted me about it. I knew she would. She asked me why I didn't like my name anymore. I felt my eyes fill with tears.

"They think I'm white, mom," I confessed, bawling.

"Who thinks you're white?

"The girls at school. They always say I sound like a white girl and now they saw dad," I blubbered.

She pulled me into her chest. I cried and apologized for crying. I felt weak, and I was so upset that I had let girls at school bring me to tears. Mom took my face in her hands and looked me in the eyes. She stared adoringly for a moment.

"Listen, for the rest of your life, you'll be too much for some people and not enough for others. But you can never abandon who you are."

She spent the next hour showering me with compliments: "You're beautiful!" "You are smart!" "You are the strongest person I know!"

She was worried that the bullying would turn physical. She knew that being in a wheelchair with extremely fragile bones would turn serious if a schoolyard fight happened. Before sending me to school the next day, she took one of my father's socks and filled it with rocks. She tied the sock around the frame of my wheelchair, down by my feet.

"You are never allowed to start a fight," she started. "But if someone puts their hands on you, you make sure you finish that fight with this."

I wasn't sure how I was going to explain this sock filled with rocks to Betty if she asked, but I went to school a little more confident that day. It wasn't that I was armed with a sock filled with rocks that made me feel confident. It was that mom reminded me of my strength. I had faced dozens of broken bones and multiple surgeries. I'd felt physical pain that no 12 year old should ever endure. Surely, I could confidently endure a few mean girls.

I knew who I was, and I knew that trying to be something that I wasn't watered down who I was and came off completely inauthentic. It was downright silly because neither Buffy nor Brooke would have felt as good as the warrior I had already proven to be. I just needed to be reminded that person was Taniya, an awkward black 12-year-old in a bright pink wheelchair.

***

During a training session at work, mom got dropped on her face while being taught a maneuver to use to subdue unruly prisoners. She broke her jaw. That would be the first and only time someone who loved me broke anything. I felt terrible for her. She couldn't chew. She could barely talk. She was on Worker's Comp while she recovered, but she never returned to work for the Suffolk County Police Department. She hated that job.

Ashley and I were older. There were more activities for her to attend: band concerts, parent-teacher conferences, dance recitals and sports practices. Things she didn't want to sleep through. Tevon was only 3 and she wanted to be as present for him as she was for Ashley and I when we were that age. My major medical needs were met, for now. I had my custom wheelchair, crutches, and walker. There were no surgeries in my immediate future. That left her a little bit more confident in giving up the extensive benefits package she had as a county employee, namely, the top-tier health insurance plan we had. She took a pay cut when she started selling insurance at our local Allstate office. The same office where I sustained my very first fracture. That broken wrist happened at a desk that was now in mom's workplace.

We had come full circle. I was 12 and at school. She was at work only feet away from where this all started.

There's Not Enough Bubble Wrap

Mom said from the start that she refused to "wrap me in bubble wrap." She knew that all my childhood activities would have to be adapted because I was disabled. I had to find a way to play with other kids. That often meant mom was standing on the side, cringing and praying that playtime always ended well. Sometimes it didn't, especially when other kids were involved. I wanted to be like other kids and was still learning my limitations.

One day, I let a neighborhood kid push me in my wheelchair.

"Faster!" I squealed with delight.

He pushed me faster and faster until I went flying out of my wheelchair and hit the concrete. I had a really bad habit of not wearing the seatbelt. I broke my hip and femur that day. After hours in the emergency room and two pretty serious fractures, mom could have refused to let me play outside with other kids. Instead, she did the opposite. She wanted me with other kids. She encouraged me to play outside.

There are many reasons why I love my mom. The biggest of them was her uncanny ability to put my growth and emotional and social needs first. She knew that all my childhood activities would help my development in a way her fear could not. Maybe that was just her selfless nature. I think it's more likely that she was intentionally trying to ensure I would be courageous, curious, and not held back by my physical limitations. Because of that, I always felt unlimited. No matter what I could or could not do, I always believed I could try, and more importantly, I had the courage to try. I always recognized the *danger* in the things I wanted to try. I just ignored the consequences because the consequences of playing were the exact same consequences from my daily life: a broken bone. I could sneeze and break my wrist or I could catch a ball and break my wrist. I knew which one sounded more fun.

***

I could only *therapy walk,* which meant I could take a few steps here and there. I could get around my house with my walker when I wanted to. Those times were few and far between, so my legs were not very strong. But I had incredible upper body strength from pushing the manual wheelchair. I never saw my poorly functioning legs as much of a hindrance because my arms made up for it.

We had a pear tree in our backyard. Ashley and I would pick pears off it and eat them in the summertime. I watched that tree grow. It was really small and skimpy on the fruit it produced. As the years went by, the tree grew exceptionally. It was tall and looked sturdy. And it produced pears quicker than Ashley and I could pick them. Sometimes we just hung out under that tree telling secrets and singing songs. One day, out of the blue, I decided I wanted to climb that tree. Mom had worked all night so she was inside sleeping. I asked Ashley to pull my wagon underneath the tree. Once she did, I stood inside the wagon.

"I'm gonna climb this tree. Watch."

Ashley, naturally fearful, looked at me like I was crazy.

Unsteady on my legs, I grabbed the lowest branch and pulled myself up. Strictly using my arms, I ascended higher and higher. Ashley watched in awe as I hung on like some deranged baby chimpanzee. Once I was satisfied with how high I had climbed, I realized I wasn't sure how I could get down. I didn't trust my legs enough to navigate me down.

"I'm stuck," I told Ashley.

Her immediate reaction was to go get mom. I begged her not to. I knew mom gave me a lot of leeway, but being stuck in a tree might be an inch too far. I thought she might never let me play outside again.

I got to the lowest branch I could find using only my arms.

"Ashley, I need help!"

I knew my sister wasn't about to climb the tree with me. *What good would that do anyway?* We'd both be stuck together in the tree.

"Let go. I'll catch you," she said, holding her arms out.

She expected that I was just going to let go and hoped to catch me. I didn't have many choices so I made her promise she wouldn't let me hit the ground. Once she did, I inhaled deeply and let go. By the grace of God, my 7-year-old sister caught me in her arms.

Later in life, I told my mom about that day and how I abandoned all fear and let myself fall out of a tree. She shook her head in disbelief and said, "You're lucky." By that point, I had already learned I wasn't lucky, I was blessed! I was blessed with a mother who was practically fearless. At times when things I did worried her, she never let it show. She most notably said, "I will not wrap her in bubble wrap!" She knew even the best safety measures wouldn't keep the fractures at bay, but they could steal my childhood. I reflect back on that time in sheer awe. I don't know how she did it. How did she say yes to activities that she knew could hurt me?

Like the day she let me join a wheelchair basketball team. I wasn't permitted to play in the school gym, but I had this insanely competitive streak. I wanted to play, but there was no getting around the liability that the schools were unwilling to take, and I couldn't exactly run, so most gym activities weren't feasible. To appease me, mom would take me to local Special Olympics events on the weekends. I hated those events! The best thing that ever came out of those was meeting a coach of a wheelchair basketball team. He asked if I wanted to join. Mom said yes before I could. I was so excited!

I was the only girl on an all-boys team. I knew nothing about basketball, except the '90s incarnation of the NBA Bulls was arguably the best basketball team to ever play. You would've thought I was Michael Jordan based on the amount of smack I talked. Dad was a huge basketball fan. I felt like I was finally doing something he could be proud of. I wanted him to brag about me to his friends. I didn't think it would happen, but secretly, that's what I wished for.

Mom and dad sat through every game with huge smiles on their faces, including the game where the opposing team had a player dubbed "the refrigerator." He was a solid-looking black high school student, and was one of the older kids on the team. He was also in a wheelchair, so that kind of leveled the playing field. I'm not going to lie, one look at him and even I questioned if I would actually come out of that game in one piece. We lost that game and pretty much every game. I don't recall us being very good. My wheelchair basketball career lasted all of one season. The appeal wore off rather quickly.

It was never about basketball or sports for me. It was about the risk of doing things that challenged other people's logic of who they thought I should be. I didn't want my wheelchair to confine me physically or mentally. I was so afraid of being forced into a box and made to stay there my whole life. I was searching for something to define myself by. I didn't want to *just* be the handicapped girl. But I wouldn't have minded being "the handicapped basketball player." I was searching for an identity based on skills, talents, and dreams. I didn't want who I was to forever be tied to my physical limitations. Without ever verbalizing that, mom just understood. She was so tuned into me that somehow she just got it.

When I wanted to try Wheelchair racing, she let me race competitively. She even hired a coach for a brief period of time. When I wanted to dance, she searched high and low and found an adaptive dance class. The only time she said no was when she didn't have the extra money to afford it. She never said no because something was dangerous or might be too difficult for me to accomplish.

When I wanted to learn how to inline skate, because that's what all the kids in the '90s were doing, she didn't remind me that I could only walk short distances with a pair of crutches.

"You save up your money, and when you have enough to afford them, I'll take you to the store and we'll get you skates," she said.

I saved every dollar I was given, and true to her word, she took me to the store and I bought a pair of black and purple rollerblades. I learned how to inline skate. Although, when you're skating and using crutches simultaneously, it looks like skiing meets ice skating. I didn't care that I wasn't moving like the other kids. I was thrilled that I was doing what other kids could do.

When I wanted to go to Space Camp, mom said yes, knowing we couldn't afford it. I dreamed of spending all summer training like an astronaut. Dad thought I was crazy. Zero gravity and astrophysics just did not sound like a good time to him. Mom knew I loved space. After all, a telescope appeared on more than one Christmas list. I think I got a total of three of them, each more high-powered than the next. I filled out the application. There was one question I wanted to skip altogether. "*Do you have any health conditions?*"

I did, but why did that matter? *Zero gravity meant zero stress on my bones. I shouldn't fracture anything.*

As much as I wanted to skip that question, there was no getting around the fact that the application required a medical form filled out by a doctor. I had to have a physical and surely my doctor was not going to lie.

When the "rejection" letter came from Space Camp, no one besides me seemed surprised. I didn't meet the requirements to attend. Did that mean I wasn't healthy enough? I wasn't capable? I wasn't strong? It didn't matter what that actually meant because it simply said, "You are *limited.*" It didn't matter how my family treated me. I had to face a world that may be unwilling to let me try. It is a world filled with restrictions and limits.

I'm not naive to the fact that I wouldn't be who I am today without who my mom was. She fortified me by refusing to limit me. I didn't know it then, but she gave me a gift that would last me a lifetime. A gift I would need to rely on heavily in adulthood.

Ties Still Bind When The Rest Falls Apart

October 31, 1993, is a day that will forever be seared in my mind. That's the day that everything I thought to be true fell apart. My parents had carefully crafted a world that was safe, secure, and comfortable. By all accounts, we were middle class. In creating that world for Ashley and I, they may have ignored the enormity of some of their problems.

My parents always had financial stress. My first 12 years of life nearly bankrupted them. Yet, they were always able to provide, but sometimes just barely. Mom never made a big deal about what she couldn't afford. She would always redirect our focus to what we already had. I'd ask for the latest Barbie accessory: car, pool, plane, or van. If it was Barbie, I had to have it.

Mom would reply coolly, "Taniya, you don't need that. You already have a Barbie house, Corvette, camper, and pool!"

Ashley and I never pushed past that point. We had a lot of things, so we knew if mom was telling us no, there was a reason. We knew that reason was financial, but we didn't ask much. Ashley now says, half-jokingly, that she didn't even know what bills were when we were kids.

Mom volunteered at our church's food pantry. Ashley and I would go with her while she put together bags of food for families to pick up. The food pantry didn't carry meat outside of canned tuna, chicken and Spam. Still, mom was meticulous in making sure those bags all contained items that could make a balanced meal: a box of stove-top stuffing, a can of corn, a pack of dinner rolls, and a gallon of milk. She quietly hoped that the family might have a pack of chicken or some ground beef to complete the food pyramid she tried to create with these bags. She'd save the *good cereal* for families with children. The Lucky Charms and Fruity Pebbles were kept to the side for the single mom with four or five kids, the same super sweet cereals we had at home that rarely appeared in the food pantry. The church food pantry always had an abundance of Cheerios though, so anybody could get those.

While we knew people from disadvantaged families, we weren't a disadvantaged family. We had extra of everything I saw stocked in the church's food pantry. We never went to bed hungry. We had more toys than we knew what to do with. We had all the love we could ask for. In fact, the home I grew up in had so much extra that my parents could foster children and begin the process of adopting a son. Most of it was great optics. My parents were great at rejoicing in public and struggling in private.

It was a damp Halloween afternoon as my bus pulled down my street. When I rode the handicapped bus, I got dropped off right in front of my house. In the distance, I could see what looked like a lot of garbage down by my mailbox. As we got closer, I noticed a lot of pink. It looked like a lot of girls' stuff, maybe Barbie stuff. I was confused as to why someone would be throwing away Barbie stuff near my house. When the bus reached my house, I recognized that it was *my* Barbie house! Ashley's was out there too. I saw the vacuum mom used on "cleaning Sundays" just lying on the lawn. Mom was nervously walking up and down the driveway. I could tell she was thinking. At the time, I thought she was as perplexed as I was about why all our belongings were strewn everywhere. Not just our toys, but also our couches, our kitchen table, TVs, lamps, and tons of bags of God only knows what. Mom wasn't confused. She knew exactly what had happened.

We'd been evicted.

She was trying to plan what to do next. She didn't say much. She put me in the car and drove down the block to pick up Ashley at the bus stop. In complete silence, we drove to Tevon's daycare to pick him up. I think I expected to get back to the house and see everything normal again, for all of our things to be back in our house. I was almost shocked when we returned and everything was still piled up on the curb. I didn't understand the concept of eviction. I couldn't grasp the idea that you could live somewhere for years and one day, someone could come in and throw all your stuff on the front lawn.

Mom started sifting through the stuff. Feeling helpless, I started looking through things too. I felt violated that some strangers had rummaged through my bedroom, touching everything that belonged to me. Things I took pride in, things my mom had worked hard to give us, were just strewn about like trash. The neighbors across the street started staring out their front window. I knew enough to be embarrassed and ashamed. Although, I didn't know why.

Mom found a bag of linens and towels. Whoever packed up our linen closet must have just emptied the whole closet into this one bag. As she started pulling the pieces out, it was in one big knot. That wasn't how mom kept her linen closet. Fitted sheets on one shelf, towels on another, and the flat sheets and pillowcases shared a shelf. She also sorted the entire closet by color. Now, it was just one big ball of fabric in a bag. She found three pillowcases and handed them to me.

"I want you guys to go trick or treat," she said.

Was she serious?

"Go ahead," she said. "I'll stay here and wait for your dad!"

She was 100% serious. Mom wouldn't let one bad moment steal any piece of childhood. We knew Tevon had never gone trick or treating. She wasn't going to deny him the opportunity to do something we had planned for weeks. Tevon was already dressed in his Spiderman costume. He wore it to daycare that morning. Ashley and I had left our costumes home. We had planned to come home from school, change, and then go trick or treating. There was no telling where those costumes were among all this stuff outside.

As kids and their parents started making their way down our block, I felt my face blush. I didn't want to be seen by somebody I went to school with. Surely being seen collecting all your worldly processions off the sidewalk would be a reason to get picked on. So I wrangled Ashley and Tevon.

"Let's go get some candy," I said.

"Be back in two hours, and don't leave this neighborhood!" She started. Then, she said something that would reverberate in my ears for the next four years. "Your dad is on his way. He should be here by the time you guys get *home.*"

We didn't have a *home* to go back to. We were now homeless. We were what homelessness in America looked like: a young family with an unfortunate set of circumstances that wiped out any opportunity to save money.

***

Once mom left the police department, money was a bit more scarce than it had been since mom wasn't making the same salary at

Allstate as she was at the police department. At Allstate, she relied heavily on her commission—a commission that was swallowed in part by medical expenses. There were always co-pays and deductibles that had to be paid. One hundred dollars just to walk into the emergency room, which I still had to do at least once a month. Another 45 dollars for a follow-up with my orthopedist. It all added up quickly.

I don't know how long they had gone without paying the rent, but knowing my mom, she thought she'd be able to make it happen. That woman pulled more than a few rabbits out of a hat. I don't know how she did it sometimes. She made things happen simply because she never allowed herself to believe they wouldn't happen. Her belief is what fueled us as a family.

***

Ashley, Tevon, and I returned with our loot. Mom and dad were sitting on the porch steps talking. They had loaded a few bags of stuff into dad's car. Just some essentials: a few toys for Tevon, dad's work uniforms, and a few pieces of clothes that she knew were already washed. She didn't want to take clothes that were dirty because where was she going to wash them?

We spent the next several hours driving around looking for a decent motel. We needed something relatively cheap, but mom would not settle for anything less than clean. She'd go to the front desk and ask what the nightly fee was. If it fit in her budget, she'd ask to see the room. The first several rooms she walked into caused her to walk back to the car looking defeated. Some of them she refused to go into because she recognized the name from the booking paperwork on some prostitutes brought to her precinct. We must have gone to ten or twelve places before she settled on the Terryville Motor Lodge in Port Jefferson. At the time, it was a seedy motel, but a lot less seedy than some of the others. The room only had two full-sized beds. Ashley and I took one. Mom, dad, and Tevon took the other. Mom didn't sleep much that night. I heard her on the phone most of the night calling family. I know she was plotting her next move.

Where were the five of us going tomorrow? What would happen to all of our stuff?

The next morning, we woke up in our new reality. Without missing a beat, mom started shouting orders.

"Brush your teeth! Wash your face! We leave in 20 minutes!" She was serious. We had one sink for five people and she wanted everyone ready to leave in 20 minutes. Thank God she showered us the night before. I kept thinking, *where does she think we're going? Were we expected to go to school?*

I was preoccupied with the events of the prior day.

Where was my stuff? Where was my dog, Chardonnay?

She was home alone the day we were evicted. There was no message or note about where she was taken. I was terrified she had gotten out the front door while our stuff was being taken out and ran away.

What if she's been hit by a car and was hurt? Was she wondering where we had gone? Why we hadn't come back for her? Was she scared?

She got scared relatively easily. She probably felt like I felt. We both woke up that morning in a place we were familiar with and comfortable in. By lunch, we were displaced, confused, and wondering *how do we get back to that comfortable place?*

I couldn't find any of my clothes in the bags mom had grabbed. I know she didn't intentionally leave my clothes behind. Everyone was such a mess, and in a rush, she somehow missed a bag that would have come out of my bedroom. All I had to wear was the same black jeans and purple T-shirt I had worn to school the day before. I hoped nobody would remember that outfit. It was fairly unassuming and muted. I doubted anyone would recognize the basic purple shirt when the halls had been filled with kids in Halloween costumes the day prior.

I knew I couldn't protest. Mom wasn't in the mood for complaints because she needed Ashley and Tevon, who were much younger, to just follow suit without having to answer questions that she didn't have the answers to. Questions like, "Where are we going?" "What happens next?" "What if the teachers find out?" "How will mom feed us dinner?" all remained unasked.

While Ashley, Tevon, and I were at school, mom collected as much as she could fit in dad's car. Those Barbie houses, TVs, stereos, and furniture all were left behind. She got some of my clothes. I was so relieved to learn I was not going to have to wear the same purple T-shirt and black jeans until I went to college.

After the first night in the motel, we relocated to Nana's house—a modest two-family home in Nassau County. Aunt D, her husband Gary, and my young cousin Cannon lived in the apartment upstairs. Nana truly didn't have the extra space to take in a family of five, but she did it anyway. We took over her living room, sleeping on her pull-out sofas. We would wake up super early and get ready for school. Mom would drive us an hour away to our schools after dropping dad off at work. She'd then head to work herself, only to have to make the same trip in reverse eight hours later. It was exhausting for her, but she did it with very little complaining.

Shortly after moving in with Nana, we lost Tevon. Mom and dad had a routine visit with Tevon's social worker and the adoption agency. They set off for New York City one morning after dropping Ashley and me off at school. They had done this many times before. It was normally just a status update of sorts. They'd make sure Tevon was still happy and healthy and explain the next steps in the adoption process to Mom and dad. I'd attended these visits before and didn't think this one was any different. Yet, it was. It was majorly different.

When mom picked us up from school that afternoon, she looked sad. I could tell something was weighing heavily on her mind. She put me in her minivan. That van was much more wheelchair-friendly than dad's car. It was easier to get my chair in and out of. So whenever mom was driving us around, she took the van. Once inside, I looked in the back to say hi to Tevon. All I saw was his winter jacket lying across the seat. My heart sank. I knew he wasn't in school. He went to the city with mom and dad.

Why wasn't he here?

"Mom, where's Tevon?" I asked, feeling like I already knew the answer.

She started to cry and muttered something about his birth mom or his previous foster mom having a *better space* for him right now. That couldn't be true. His previous foster mom was not planning on adopting him. We were. She had five kids of her own and two foster kids. *How could she have better space?* His birth mom was a drug addict. Tevon was born addicted to crack. Certainly, neither of them could offer Tevon more than my family could. Then it hit me. Yes, they could. We didn't have anything anymore!

Mom jumped into part explanation and part rant about how she wouldn't stand for this. She was going to get him back. She already saw herself as his mother. She just needed the adoption to be finalized. She said she'd get a lawyer. I don't know if she believed what she was saying. *Who was she kidding?* We couldn't afford a lawyer, nor did she have a leg to stand on. Let's face it, adoption agencies aren't in the business of placing kids with homeless parents.

The more she spoke, the more the reality of our new situation settled in. In one week, everything I knew fell apart. My circumstances were different. My family was different. We were back to being just a family of four in one day. Everybody was reeling and hurting, but we didn't talk about it. I learned how good my parents were at suppressing their feelings. They just continued to move through daily life as if everything was exactly the same, while they knew it wasn't.

I was gripped by emotions I couldn't explain. I was hurt. I was angry. I was afraid. I was terrified that if anyone found out my parents couldn't keep a roof over our heads, Ashley and I would also be removed and most likely separated. The thought of having to manage life without Ashley seemed impossible. I was also worried that if people found out, they would look at my parents differently. I was too young to understand that not all homelessness in America looked like a dirty man with unwashed hair begging for spare change. I didn't want my parents to feel bad, like they had failed their children. I was old enough to understand what I had cost them. They were hard-working people who were dealt a hand they were wholly unprepared for. There are no savings when every dollar goes to medical expenses.

***

Even though it was now just the four of us, Nana's house couldn't accommodate us. Ashley and I were loud kids used to having a whole house to run through and leave a trail of Barbies. While living at Nana's, mom made sure we picked up behind ourselves and kept our noise level down. The four of us were sharing two pull-out couches with thin mattresses. Not the most comfortable sleeping quarters, but we were together. Mom and dad would disappear in the middle of the night to Nana's bathroom to have sex. No kid wants to think of their parents having sex, so it really freaked me out when they came walking back from the bathroom hand-in-hand with messy hair. Those nights were just awkward. I wouldn't make eye contact with either of them until the next day.

Nana's house was also way too far from mine and Ashley's schools. That one hour in the morning rush hour traffic got us there late every day. Mom and dad both knew we needed to go somewhere else, but they didn't have a plan. It's hard to figure out how to get back on your feet when you never expected to be knocked off them in the first place. I knew my mom had the fortitude to get us back. I just didn't know how long it would take her.

Conveniently Inconvenient

My maternal grandfather was in the early stages of Alzheimer's Disease. It was a disease that my mom was terrified of developing in her old age. She had watched her own grandmother succumb to the disease and die. Knowing it was inherited, she worried about getting it. When her father was diagnosed with early onset Alzheimer's in his sixties, she wanted to be near him. She wanted to spend time with him, but I think some part of her wanted to watch the disease progression in an effort to be prepared for a disease she was convinced was coming for her. She also needed somewhere to live, somewhere that would put her closer to the schools Ashley and I went to.

Mom told grandma that we could stay with her and grandpa. Mom could offer grandma help with what she needed most: caring for grandpa. In turn, mom could have what she needed most: a comfortable place for her family to live. Grandma was adamant about not putting grandpa in a nursing home. She wanted to care for him herself. That was dangerous for her. She was a tiny five-foot-tall woman. Grandpa was easily over six feet, and an avid gun and knife collector with an affinity for old war movies. The more the disease ravaged his brain, the less he saw his wife when he looked at my grandma and the more he saw a threat.

Grandma wasn't thrilled with that idea, but she wasn't opposed to it either. Grandma loved to care for people. Maybe even more than my mom did. We couldn't visit Grandma without her trying to feed us a full meal. She would start listing menu options the minute people walked through the door like she ran a restaurant and those were the daily specials.

"You want a cheeseburger and fries? How about some chicken salad? I've got tuna too. What about some bacon and eggs?" For every no she was given, she would just call out another dish. Most people would eventually concede and just eat something.

Grandma did make the best cheeseburgers.

We moved in just after Christmas. Things were almost immediately contentious. My grandfather hated my dad. He truly believed my mom was too good for him. There was nothing in the world that would make him forget that. So dad didn't come with us. He settled in with Nana again. That wasn't anything new to him. Every time he and mom would "split up," that's where he'd go. I was okay with that. My relationship with dad was more strained than ever. I was filled with teenage angst that every girl around that age gets. I was angry that my life, as I knew it, had been completely disrupted. *Had I not endured enough in childhood to have earned the right to some semblance of normalcy?* I was mad, and because dad and I didn't have a good relationship to begin with, he was the low-hanging fruit. It was easy to be mad at him. His absence stressed Ashley a bit, but we were busy with school and reunited on the weekends.

Mom didn't want to change our schools. She thought that it might be too traumatic. So she drove us to school every day and picked us up after work, and we headed back to grandma and grandpa's. It was as normal as we could get at the moment. I was just excited to sleep in a real bed.

Grandpa was a surly old man who did not envision spending his retirement having his adult daughter and grandchildren living with him. He made that abundantly clear more than once. Mom remained unfazed by his complaints. She had a stern resolve that this wouldn't last forever, but because it was our current situation, we would just hunker down and make the best of it. So that's exactly what we did.

A Fresh Start

Grandma and grandpa lived in a quiet little town on Long Island. Mount Sinai had a small population and a median household annual income of $142,000. That tells you everything you need to know about Mount Sinai. It was not a very diverse town. I'm not sure what brought my very black grandparents to a predominantly white town decades earlier. I can only imagine my Virginia-born-and-raised grandmother stuck out like a sore thumb at the local grocery store.

My mom got the brilliant idea to enroll us in school there. We would be able to take the bus. She had heard great things about the school. It was a "Blue Ribbon" school with enough money for arts and sports programs. On paper, it was the school every parent would want their kid to go to. It checked all of mom's boxes. But it left the socioeconomic box completely blank.

At Longwood, we were middle class and kids still gave me hell. We were now homeless, so I would definitely be considered poor in Mount Sinai schools. You couldn't drive down any of the gorgeous tree-lined streets without seeing fancy cars and big houses. I knew there would be no way in hell the poor black girl in the wheelchair would fit in. Initially, I didn't want to go, but the more I thought about it, the more I liked the sound of changing schools. I thought that I would just be able to ditch those pesky special education classes. Nobody in Mount Sinai knew me. They didn't know my history. I'd be able to reinvent myself as the kid I wanted to be seen as: the smart, talented, capable kid who has a bright future in front of her. Mount Sinai was going to give me that opportunity.

Wrong!

What I got was more of the same. That "Blue Ribbon" school gave me more of what I'd always gotten, an "education" devoid of any real challenge. They gave me no preliminary testing to at least pretend they were interested in seeing what I was capable of. No, they saw what everyone else saw: "a girl in a wheelchair." I couldn't wrap my mind around how that image was synonymous with dumbness. Before I even got to open my mouth, school administrators already believed I would be unable to hold my own in regular classes. It was a stigma I just couldn't shake off. *If a new school wasn't going to give me a chance, who would?*

I wanted the opportunity to succeed or fail on my own accord. I didn't want to be successful because I coasted through life never being challenged academically. OI may have stolen some physical facets of my life, but it didn't steal my dreams. Not many people asked, but those who dared to ask what I wanted to be knew I had dreams of being an astronaut. Maybe I wasn't cut out for Space Camp. Maybe, physically, I could not be an astronaut. The lack of gravity in space reduces bone density. As a kid with Brittle Bone Disease, I couldn't afford to lose any bone density.

My second top career choice was a doctor—specifically, an orthopedic surgeon. I wanted to set fractures, perform surgeries, and lead research that would eventually cure this unforgiving disease. That meant I wanted to go to college. I knew that in order to get into medical school, I needed to be competitive. That meant real classes and really good grades. I wanted somebody besides my mom to believe in me. It is so incredibly hard to hold on to any ounce of self-worth when everyone I met led the conversation with doubt.

At the very least, I wanted to learn real science. That was my favorite subject. I had a telescope, microscope, and multiple chemistry sets, all of which were Christmas gifts. I was a true nerd. Because I loved science so much, I thought I could immediately excel in it and use that as leverage to negotiate my way out of Special Ed. Mom and I met with some administrators and members of the guidance department. I didn't have an official Individualized Educational Plan. It's a plan made for students with special needs. It takes into consideration any reasonable accommodations that are needed. Mom always seemed to just show up to the school with a list of demands every year. I never had anything in writing. Mt. Sinai just fell in line and agreed with what was done at my previous school. The thing that stood out most in that meeting was that everyone refused to talk to me. They directed all questions and comments to mom.

I was so used to people not directing questions to me, but it felt different this time. I was 14 years old, headed into a new high school, and the people who would be responsible for my education wouldn't even recognize me as a person. They definitely didn't care what I wanted to learn. I was seething as the minutes passed. I heard mom consent to extra time on tests. When you're in Special Ed, they automatically assume it will take you longer to take tests. They agreed to allow me to leave class three minutes before the bell rang, giving me extra time to get to the next class. That was as much a logistical issue as a safety concern. When you have to wait for the elevator, it can take longer than just taking the stairs, which isn't an option in a wheelchair. God help you if the janitor had to bring something down to the basement. You could wait forever! Also, this schedule kept me from changing classes with a mass of rushing teenagers, running, skipping or just not looking where they were going and knocking me over. Truthfully, I posed my own risk to those kids. I ran over quite a few toes in those halls.

I agreed with all the logistical stuff. No contact sports, fine! I would only be assigned a bottom locker? You got it! Leave class early? I was on board with that too. However, I had one non-negotiable. I refused a one-on-one aide. I didn't need it. I could stand and walk, so transferring from my chair to the toilet was not an issue. Once I got through puberty, my fractures subsided a lot. Needing someone to keep me safe wasn't as necessary as it was in grade school. I could write on my own and push my own chair. To be honest, I just didn't want to be followed around all day by an adult. Like most 14-year-old kids, I wanted independence. If I heard anybody in that meeting say aide, I was fully prepared to fight that.

I hadn't said much the whole meeting. When they finished with their checklist, I piped up.

"Give me science," I said."Please just let me take regular science." My voice was weak when I asked.

I was mad at myself for not being more forceful, but I knew I was going to be shot down.

But I wasn't—at least not immediately.

"Let us talk it over with the science teacher and see what he thinks," the guidance counselor said. "Mainstream science is hard."

What led her to believe I was unprepared for hard? Everything in life was hard. I struggled to just go to the bathroom. I wasn't asking for easy. I didn't want easy.

"If it's too hard, I'll go back."

I knew I had no intentions of quitting. That wasn't my nature, but I felt like I had to offer them an out because it was clear they were convinced I was going to fail.

"We'll see!" she said, placating me.

I doubt she ever asked. She told me weeks after I started school that the science teacher declined to have me in his class. He felt I was too far behind and wouldn't be able to keep up.

I doubt I ever had true allies in the public school administration. I had a bunch of adults that only wanted to protect me because I was a liability. When people won't even acknowledge your personhood, it's pretty clear they certainly aren't interested in your feelings. I wanted to be angry, but I was too tired to be outraged. I was so tired of trying to prove myself. I felt like no matter what I did, there would always be a huge faction of people who would refuse to believe in me. Perhaps school administrators were always going to be among them.

When I started Mt. Sinai, it was already February. The school year was more than half over. The only thing more awkward than being the new kid was being the new kid who comes in more than halfway through the year. The kids were nice, at best. At worst, they were simply indifferent to my presence.

The only way I could have stuck out more is if I were from a different country. I was one of only a handful of black students and one of only two wheelchair users. I looked around at first and thought, *what the hell am I doing here?* I didn't look like them, I didn't move like them, and I wasn't even allowed to take classes with them. I was 14 and a little over three feet tall.

***

In middle school, I had seen a television interview with Dominique Moceanu, a gymnast who would go on to compete as part of the USA Gymnastics team in the 1996 Summer Olympics. I became fascinated with her as I watched her speak. There was no doubt that she was talented. What stood out to me was she was around my age and very tiny. I remember my mom telling me that because of the way gymnasts train, and the fact that most of them start really young, they tend to be short girls. I still don't know if that's true, but that became my go-to lie. Anytime someone asked why I was so short, I'd tell them I took gymnastics as a kid. I was in a wheelchair, unable to walk, but naively expected people would believe I was a gymnast. No one ever questioned it, which is why I stuck with it.

***

Something about these kids seemed different. I almost knew that lie wasn't going to work here. I worried about what questions people would ask and how I would answer them. I wanted to be seen. I have a huge personality, but in childhood, I spent so much time trying to blend into the background because standing out meant being looked at. People would openly gawk at me. I always felt like I was on display and knew no matter how uncomfortable I was, it was expected that I would be nice. How do you make friends if you're not nice? How do you remain nice when you are incredibly uncomfortable? You learn how to be funny.

Since I always had to be *on* because I always had an audience, I became quite the comedian. I'm still the funniest person I know. I often was the muse for my own material: cracking short jokes and poking fun at my disability. I stopped just shy of being disparaging. If you can make people laugh *with* you, they are not laughing *at* you. If I could make it a joke first, no one could weaponize it and use it to hurt me. That got me through middle school. I wasn't sure it was going to work at Mount Sinai, though. I questioned if I had what it took to actually go to school there.

Being such a small town, most of those kids had known each other since Kindergarten. They shared the same classes throughout school. It was very cliquey. Maybe it was just being 14 or maybe it was that I had come from a school where kids hated me just for speaking, but I didn't want to fade into the background anymore. I wanted friends—lots of friends. I wanted to stand out for something. I desperately wanted to be liked.

I knew that was a tall order because in hallways filled with designer clothes, I didn't have much. The only coat I had was a school jacket from Longwood. A dark green coat with white leather sleeves emblazoned with a huge "L" on the front and "Longwood" across the back. I wanted that jacket so badly when they were sold in middle school. I remember bringing the order form home and asking mom if I could order one. It was 90 dollars. I knew we didn't have that type of money. To my surprise, mom said yes and filled out the order form. When she handed it back to me with a check, I knew she was pulling that money from someplace else.

Was she going to skip lunch for the month? Only buy the necessities at the grocery store and skip the overpriced snacks? Not buy herself new shoes for work?

I knew she would do something to make up for that 90 dollars. Because I knew the sacrifice involved, that jacket was my favorite possession. It was also February in New York. Not wearing a jacket was not an option. I never thought of the implications of wearing a rival school's jacket to my current school—it really wasn't a good look.

During one of my first days at Mt. Sinai, Mr. Kulik, the math teacher who doubled as the football coach, was behind me as I rolled through the front doors.

"We're going to have to get you a new jacket!" he said.

He wasn't mocking me. How could he be? He had no way of knowing that I had just lost everything. I only still had this jacket because I wore it to school the day of the eviction. There was no malice in that statement. Just the stark reality that I had this huge secret that no one would ever understand. Therefore, no one could ever know.

I made a core group of friends but didn't let anybody too close. I couldn't see my friends outside of school. People surmised that my parents were overprotective, and that's why I didn't invite them over. The truth was, where could I invite them to? I had a secret that I had to protect. There was a roof over my head, but I was technically homeless.

"My parents are *weird,*" I told people. My friends assumed that meant they were strict and didn't allow me to have much of a social life. I didn't do anything to correct that perception of my parents. There was no way to explain it. Them being strict or overprotective sounded like a good excuse!

I met Alex during my first week at school. We were in the same gym class. Being in gym class was a completely new experience. I never got to participate in gym at Longwood. If I wasn't getting physical therapy, I was spending the period in the library researching athletes to write essays on because that was a safe activity for the girl with Brittle Bone Disease. I could tell you more about Kristi Yamaguchi, Magic

Johnson, and Mary Lou Retton by eighth grade than any ESPN biographer ever could.

Alex was approachable. She was one of the first girls I saw not surrounded by a large group of other girls. It was much easier to approach one girl and be rejected than it was to be rejected by a larger group of popular girls following each other around like a flock of geese.

Alex was so warm, and she didn't ask any questions, which was a relief. She was one of the first people who didn't make me feel like an outsider. We quickly became friends. I had a carefully guarded secret, and she made that easier to keep. Alex didn't *need* to be invited over. She was not permitted to go out on Fridays. Alex is Jewish and in observance of Shabbat, her mother required her to be home by sundown on Friday nights. I'd complain about my "strict parents" and she'd understand. She quickly became my best friend. Her house was within walking distance of the school. We'd walk there after school and I'd stay until mom picked up dad and Ashley. It was the only time I didn't have to ask mom to drop me off somewhere and drive around aimlessly until I was done.

Alex was the first person I called when I got off the bus at grandma's house. I would block grandma's number because I never wanted her to try and call me back.

Grandma would always ask me, "Didn't you just see her? What more could you have to tell her?"

Dad often echoed that sentiment.

I wanted to say, "I'm a homeless black girl in a wheelchair at this school where I don't fit in at all! This girl doesn't treat me like an *other.* I'll talk to her nine times a day if I want to!"

Everyone needs a friend like Alex. She became like a second sister to me. Alex knew all my secrets… at least all the ones I could tell her. She never knew I had nowhere to call home.

We'll Give You A Home

My grandfather was becoming more agitated with us as his disease progressed. The strain of not having her entire family under one roof was bothering my mom. She rarely complained, but I could see the worry in her eyes. She worried about dad. She worried about the future. What impact would this have on Ashley and me? We had a roof over our heads, but it didn't feel like a *home.* We knew we were guests in someone else's house. She'd say things like, "Don't make too much noise or you'll disturb grandpa," or, "Skip the music videos on MTV and watch Judge Judy with grandma while she cooks your family dinner." While I loved my grandparents very much, I never felt *at home.*

I don't know what the straw that broke the proverbial camel's back was, but mom decided that after a few short months, we would move out of her parents' house. We took up longer residence at a motel located on a busy highway. It looked like any other budget motel: two queen-sized beds, a dresser, one bathroom, and a single sink. To say it was too close for comfort is an understatement of the century. *Temporary,* they called it. The problem with temporary is that there was no definitive end date.

I was a girl trying to navigate my way into womanhood while sleeping in the same bed with my younger sister and sharing a bathroom with my dad. When I'd get my period, I'd nervously wrap my used sanitary napkins in toilet paper before throwing them away in the only garbage can, which was located outside of the bathroom. Everything had to be commingled because there wasn't enough space for four individuals. One morning, I was getting ready for school and I pulled my bra out of the top drawer. It was tangled up with a pair of dad's underwear. They were both clean. Everything in that drawer was clean. Still, I was disgusted. I wasn't a spoiled or entitled kid. But I knew I at least deserved my own drawer.

I threw myself into school because I didn't know what else to do. I couldn't go *home* every day, sit on a bed next to Ashley, and just stare at our parents. At best, we'd compromise on a primetime television show and watch it on the only TV in the room. Normally, my dad would control the programming. He was a huge fan of "Cops," the "WWF," and TMC movies. Not exactly a teenage girl's dream television lineup.

When other kids my age were watching "The Real World" and "TRL," MTV's music video countdown show, I was just praying I wasn't going to have to watch another old western.

I joined every club there was: environmental club, yearbook club, photography club, computer club, and chorus. I did them all. On days that I didn't have a club to go to, I stayed in the library for hours. I would pour over books and magazines. I was doing two things. First, I was avoiding going home, which I certainly didn't want to do. I also was trying hard to be seen as a nerd. I thought if the teachers, principal, and administrators saw me with my nose always in a book and in every club there was to join, I'd somehow shift their perception of me. I wanted people to view me in that way because in my mind, a nerd was synonymous with smart. Looking back, I know I truly believed that if I changed the preconceived notions people had surrounding my capabilities, that would be all I needed to get out of Special Ed.

Johnathan Babcock, my chorus teacher, would make me an offer that would change the trajectory of my life. One afternoon, he saw me wandering the halls aimlessly. I didn't have a club to go to that day. He knew me from chorus, but didn't *know* me. Yet, he was incredibly sensitive to me as a wheelchair user in chorus. The chorus room was not accessible, as it had elevated seating. When I joined chorus, he had to redo the seating so that I could sit with my fellow altos without being in the furthest corner of the room because I couldn't get up the steps. When we had concerts, I couldn't stand on the risers. I'd line my wheelchair at the very end of the riser. During concert rehearsals, he always checked to make sure I could see him conducting. He recognized that I was lower than all the other students. My line of sight was not the same. I felt like out of everybody at that school, he was the first person to actually *see* me.

He saw me rolling up and down in the band hallway. He couldn't have known this, but I was trying to figure out what to do. I didn't want to leave school, but because I didn't have a club, I didn't have anything to do. Usually, I'd just sit in the library. For whatever reason, I didn't feel like doing that this day. I heard someone call my name. I turned around and Mr. Babcock stood in the doorway of the chorus room.

"I have rehearsal in the auditorium in a little while. You should come!" he said.

I didn't know why he was asking, but I felt invited. Before that moment, I had felt like an outsider in school. Not only did I not feel included, but I didn't even feel wanted. Outside of the handful of friends I had, most kids there didn't make an effort to get to know me.

Being in the Special Ed class only furthered the divide between the other kids and myself. Special Ed was legal segregation. I stayed in one classroom with the same twelve kids. I wasn't in classes with 95% of the students in my grade. They didn't dislike me. They just didn't know me. It's easy to underestimate how valuable and necessary the social component of school is. Sometimes, well-meaning adults planning for, and taking care of, the special needs of a disabled child forget we also have very normal needs too.

I went to Mr. Babcock's rehearsal for the spring musical *Oklahoma*, and every show after that. The theater was a completely different world than I was used to. I didn't feel like I had to constantly prove my worth. I wanted to learn about stage lighting. Mr. Babcock made sure someone showed me the light board. I wanted to learn set construction, so they invited me to build and paint after school. Nobody questioned if I could. They were willing to just let me try. All I ever asked was for people to let me try.

Rehearsals ran into the evenings, so that was an added bonus. Mom would pick me up from rehearsal, we'd head back to the motel, where she would feed me whatever fast food she could get us for dinner. After that, I'd go to sleep knowing I could do it all again the next day. Disappearing into the fantastical world of musical theater was a much-needed distraction from my real life. One of the senior girls, Courtney, was in every show.

"This is my family," she said to me, referring to her frequent cast members. "The theater is like a home."

She had no clue how true those words would become for me as well. The theater was the only place I could go to find refuge. The only parties I ever got invited to in high school were cast parties. But those cast parties were everything to me. I finally had an identity that did not revolve around my disability. I was a "Theater Kid." Not a disabled theater kid, just a theater kid.

Let Me Out

Armed with newfound confidence, I requested a meeting with the principal. I was about to finish ninth grade. I played by the rules they set. I took their Special Ed classes. I maintained good grades. I participated in every extracurricular activity there was. Yet, my educational needs were not met. By everyone's standards, I was a successful student making honor roll. That was no grand achievement. I was being taught at least one grade level behind. I knew no one had a plan to free me of Special Ed. As far as I was concerned, it made no sense for me to be in school. I wasn't being challenged. I wasn't satisfied with the idea that this would be the remainder of my academic career. I was okay with being underestimated, but I was not okay with being treated like I was stupid. Mr. Walters, the Principal, agreed to a meeting with me and mom to discuss the plan for next year.

I spent weeks crafting a well thought out argument as to why I should be let out of Special Ed. I practiced everything I was going to say in my head. I knew I had excellent grades. I was an honor student in Special Ed. What's the worst that would happen if they let me take regular classes? I'd be average? That didn't sound like a bad deal to me. At the time, I probably would have given anything to be average.

Mr. Walters spoke and I just saw his lips moving. I didn't register anything he was saying because I knew it was another slew of excuses as to why I should remain in Special Ed. He kept circling back to "but you're doing so well." That was the point I was trying to make. I was excelling at a seventh or eighth grade curriculum as a high school freshman. Why was that commendable? While my peers were reading *Of Mice and Men* or *Romeo and Juliet*, I was doing sentence structure for the billionth time. And this guy thought it was good that I was "doing well." How could I *not* do well? I didn't have a learning disability. The more he spoke, the more annoyed I got.

This meeting was going nowhere fast. Again, the adults didn't want to listen to me.

"If you won't let me out, I'll drop out!" I blurted out in the most impulsive manner.

I knew damn well Deborah Faulk wasn't going to stand for me dropping out of high school. She shot me a quick look and I knew I better revise and justify that proclamation.

"It's a waste of time for me to come here five days a week and not learn anything," I rephrased.

Mr. Walters looked at me and blinked—*a lot.* I could tell I was starting to get through, but it wasn't totally resonating with him. I knew I had to ramp up my argument. I had to stop trying to prove myself worth, and instead make the school prove itself.

"What's the point of going to a good school if you won't give me a good education?" I asked.

It was a genuine question, but I knew that it contained just enough manipulation to win this argument. They prided themselves in being a "Blue Ribbon" school with an extremely low dropout rate. I could see him coming around. He wasn't fully on my side yet, but he was getting there. I knew if he had some assurance that I wouldn't be so out of my depth and unable to reverse course he'd get on board.

"Look, I don't want to fail. If I can't handle it, I'll be the first to say so and go back to the Special Ed classes," I offered up.

Finally, Mr. Walters gave me the first signs of some concession. He leaned back in his chair and stopped blinking so much. He agreed to one class a year. If I could maintain my grades and the pace of the course work each year, they would add an additional class with the goal of having fully mainstreamed by senior year. That was much slower than I wanted it to go, but it was more than what I had, so I conceded.

I got science first. Mainstream biology was a dream realized. I was in tenth grade and for the first time ever, I felt challenged academically. It definitely was harder. For the first time, I had to study. That in itself is a skill set I didn't have. I kept my grades up and they gave me English next. I'd get so excited right after midterms when I had to pick my classes for next year. That's when they would tell me the next mainstream class that I would get.

My circumstances at home weren't conducive to studying, writing papers, or reading. One year just bled into the next. We were still in the motel. With each changing season, I'd wonder if this was when we get to move out. It just wasn't happening. Between the weekly rates my parents paid to stay at the motel and the cost of eating out three times a day because there was no way to cook, the cost was expensive. My parents saved whatever extra they could. It just wasn't enough. They were living paycheck to paycheck.

It didn't matter what the rest of my life looked like. No one knew and no one cared. I promised I could keep up, and that's what I had to do. Too many people were expecting me to fail. It was a strange feeling because I felt like I had no room to falter. I always thought every test grade that wasn't an A was a reason to question if I could handle a mainstream course load. I was terrified at any moment they could take it away from me. There were times when I cried over test grades because they could be that detrimental to me. I was constantly in a state of having to prove myself. I don't know how I made it through four years of high school because I was a neurotic mess. My self-worth was at an all time low.

I wasn't the "pretty" girl. I was awkward and funny looking. I had prayed to be in class with these kids, and the minute I was, I felt so out of place not academically but socially. That was almost acceptable because I was a "theater nerd." I was social and outgoing, but I just never fit fully or felt like one of them. Looking back, I'm not so sure that was a bad thing. I already knew I didn't fit in, I saw no point in trying. So I was able to avoid the pitfalls of peer pressure many high school students succumb to.

By senior year, with graduation looming, I still felt like I had something to prove. My grades were good. I was fully mainstreamed and I wanted to shout from the rooftops, "I told you so!" I wanted to take a victory lap of sorts. I could walk just enough to make me fairly independent in small spaces. In class, I'd get out of my chair and sit in a regular desk. I never walked through the hallways though. I always used my wheelchair in stores and most public spaces, but I was capable of walking unaided. For whatever reason, I got the idea that walking in the graduation procession was going to be my "victory lap." For me, it was symbolic. I was going to *walk* into the future free of everything that had defined me my entire life. No more Special Ed. No wheelchair. Even if only for a single moment I wanted to redefine myself. On some level, I'm sure I also wanted to prove to people that I could do it. Perpetually proving myself was the entire theme of my high school experience. Why wouldn't I be compelled to prove myself at graduation?

Administrative red tape required that I get permission to do it. I found that a bit excessive. I just wanted to walk, a luxury afforded to all my peers. I wasn't trying to attempt flame-throwing at the ceremony. I really didn't get all the fuss over it. But as requested, I got the okay from the principal. The most interesting part was that he was a man who spent four years trying to talk me out of wanting to be in mainstream classes yet it took no coercing to get his blessing to walk during graduation. I completely expected to have to fight for that. I didn't. He didn't even point out the reality that I had never walked through the school, let alone from the school to the football field where graduation would take place. Somehow, that reality escaped me entirely.

In the days leading up to graduation, mom took me to buy a dress and shoes. I picked a long fitted blue lace dress. I normally was a jeans and T-shirt type girl, but I loved the opportunity to dress up. I picked out a pair of black, scrappy platform sandals. They were perfect for the dress and I loved them. There was just one problem. I have children's-size feet. The smallest size these sandals came in was a women's size five. I bought them anyway. I don't know what I was thinking. I was going to walk the longest distance I've ever walked at one time and I was going to do so in sandals three or four sizes too big. There is nothing like teenage idealism to make you completely blind to reality. I rationalized that while I might fall flat on my face, I was going to look good doing it.

The night before graduation, mom stayed up until the wee hours of the morning hemming my dress and graduation gown by hand. We'd come full circle. She was hemming the high school graduation gown for the kid she was told wouldn't live to see her 10th birthday. I'd come a long way. I wish in the moment I had allowed myself to acknowledge and appreciate how far I had come. I didn't. Instead, I could only see how far I had to go: college, career, walk independently, husband, family. I wanted it all. I didn't truly believe I could have it all, but I knew I wanted it.

As my classmates assembled for the procession, the energy was palpable. I inhaled deeply taking in a mix of adrenaline and excitement. I took a moment, closed my eyes and prayed quickly. I asked God to not let me start this walk and be unable to finish. I knew I had to commit to this. There was no stepping out of line to rest. It wasn't a short walk, and I knew that. I knew I was pushing the boundaries of what I physically could do. I had never walked that far. Something about pushing my limits fortified me. I made that slow and not-so-steady walk from the school to the football field and across the stage. In front of my family and peers, I accepted my high school diploma standing on my feet as an honor student. That was a reality I had envisioned since elementary school. I visualized a reality for myself, that nobody but my mom believed in.

What I hadn't planned for was having to walk back to my wheelchair, which I left in the school. I was exhausted. My legs were shaking with fatigue. For a split second I regretted making that walk because I felt like I was "failing" in the home stretch. I didn't want to cap this day off with a defeat, but I couldn't take another step. I was seconds away from sitting down on the grass until my legs stopped shaking and I had the energy to stand back up. One of my classmates, Rob, who knew me fairly well, stopped and in a moment of honest compassion offered me a piggyback ride.

"You need a ride?" he said as he crouched down next to me.

I looked at him hesitantly. I was torn between giving up or having to sit on the football field alone until my fatigue abated. I didn't want to feel like I was giving up, but I literally could not take another step. I reminded myself that the goal was to walk in the graduation procession. I had just done that. I had accomplished something that moments before it happened I was second guessing. I reached the goal. There would always be another goal, something to strive for, another time to push past my limits, but in this moment I needed help. I sucked it up, jumped on Rob's back, and thew my arms around his neck and reminded myself that this is not what defeat looks or feels like. I was so tired because I made my body do something it had never done. I was damn proud that! In that moment, I realized it's okay to need help. We all need help at times.

Accepting help is not the same as giving up.

One person who was notably absent from my graduation was Nana. While I was in high school, she was diagnosed with lung cancer.

She fought valiantly but in my junior year she passed away. I thought about her that day. I knew she would be proud. I could almost hear her shouting “hot digitty dog!” from the bleachers as I walked across the stage. That was her favorite expression to let people know that in her eyes they did well. It could be a triple word score in a game of Scrabble, an “A” on a test or getting the answer to one of her riddles. She was one of the strongest women I knew, second only to my mother. Watching her fight cancer was an almost daily reminder of the courage that is a part of my lineage. I came from a long line of women who reminded me that I was not born to fall apart. I knew that, even if I didn’t always believe it.

To be honest, I didn’t always believe it.

Girl, Get Your Head Right

I applied to colleges late. I didn't start applying until senior year. To be honest, I was exhausted. I had spent my entire academic career trying to prove I was smart enough. Did I really want to do that again with an admissions committee? I didn't. But did I want to be the girl from a small town on Long Island who never did anything else? That's what everyone had expected of me. My desire to defy that expectation was stronger than any trepidation I may have had. I dreamed that one day I could walk into Mt. Sinai High School with my college degree and shake the principal's hand to say, "Thank you for reluctantly believing in me" and "I told you so" at the same time.

It was no longer *if* I could go to college. It was *where* I would go. I was set on going away, and going far away. I had no interest in going to any of the acclaimed state universities. I wanted a new start where no one knew me. I wanted to define who I was to the world. In my mind, that meant fleeing from everyone who knew me as "the girl in the wheelchair." I wanted to leave the state. I wanted to carve out my place in this world.

I applied to UCLA, USC, UCF, Flagler College, Pepperdine University, and Notre Dame. As the rejection letters mounted, my self-confidence plummeted. I knew I didn't have the academic capital to get into any of those schools. The public school system cheated me out of that. I naively thought I made up enough work during senior year to be a viable candidate. I'd been conditioned to believe that if I wanted something bad enough, I could have it if I worked hard. After all, I'd defied all the odds to this point.

With each rejection letter, I was filled with more self-doubt. I questioned everything I thought I knew about myself. I thought about giving up. I wanted to give up. But defeat felt like I was beaten. Giving up felt like I didn't even try, which sounded slightly worse. I had only felt defeated because I was trying to live a narrative that had been written for me. A story about a girl who has to *fight* for everything. The story of an 18-year-old whose entire self-worth was tied to how smart people thought she was. The rest of my life would only be defined by kindergarten through 12th grade if I let it. At what point do I get to stop fighting against something? I did not want to spend the rest of my life overcoming stigmas, opinions, stereotypes and statistics. I wanted to finally just live a life where my success was not a surprise to people anymore. I didn't want to be an honors student because the school believed I was only smart enough for Special Ed. I didn't want to feel compelled to walk because doctors said I never would. I wanted to stop having to prove myself and my abilities.

No one was going to do that for me. I needed time. I needed to fix my thinking, rebuild my self-esteem, and determine who I wanted to be. I was trying to rewrite my narrative. In reality, I needed to rid myself of the narrative written for me and start a new story. I knew I couldn't do that with my head filled with all the messages of unworthiness that were force-fed to me by the public school system. I needed to clear my head. That meant I needed to take a break from school.

When I announced I was going to take a gap year, not a single person spared me the "You'll never go back" speech. I'm glad I had to listen to that speech. The best way to ensure I'll do something is to tell me I can't or won't do it. I then become determined in my resolve to do it. My mom wasn't thrilled with this decision, but she was supportive. When I explained to her that I doubted what I was capable of, she understood. All my childhood idealism had been replaced with tremendous self-doubt. I promised her I would go, but I wanted time to believe in myself again. She agreed. Her only stipulation was that I get a full time job. She knew me well enough to recognize my sense of self-worth was always connected to me doing something. She knew if I didn't wake up every day with something to do that I'd lose all motivation. It would be counterproductive to what I was trying to achieve.

My planned gap year turned into two. During this time, I worked for a 401(k) record keeper. Mom was in a supervisory position there and got me the job. I processed distribution requests, handled incoming calls for the distribution department, and performed basic administrative tasks. It wasn't the best job in the world, but it put gas in my car, gave me health insurance, and spending money. I knew it wasn't what I wanted to do for the rest of my life. That was a truly interesting observation because I didn't know what I wanted to do with my life anymore. When you grow up with a disability, people rarely ask you what you want to be when you grow up, as if you're expected to be a disabled child your entire life. Those who are brave enough to ask don't even let you finish before they've compiled a list of all the obstacles you'll face. It wasn't so much a matter of what I wanted to do. It was what I would be able to do. In the late '90s and at the start of the new millennium, it was common to just get a degree. It didn't matter what that degree was in. As long as you had a degree, you were automatically worth more than someone who only had a high school diploma and thus would be nearly guaranteed to secure a "good" job. I was a space camp "reject" because of my disease. So I was certain that NASA would not want me. I abandoned my dream of med school. Representation matters. I never saw a doctor in a wheelchair. I never saw anyone in health care who looked or moved like me. So when my uncle said things like, "You need to stand up to perform surgery," I internalized that. Every time a teacher said, "Med school is hard" or "You need to get good grades," it preyed on my concerns over what I lacked academically. I was acutely aware of my obstacles, but it seemed as if anytime I saw the possibilities, outsiders only saw problems.

I thought back to my days with Mr. Babcock and the theater. It was something I loved and the one thing in all my years of school I was never made to doubt. It was something I was good at, interested in, and welcomed into.

If all I needed was a degree, why not get a degree in the one thing I didn't doubt?

I didn't know what I could do with a theater degree. I didn't necessarily think I could be an actress. Not that I didn't have the talent, but when the world's greatest plays were written, they did not include Little People, and disabled people barely registered in the consciousness of playwrights. Nonetheless, a degree in theater was appealing. I could do what I love. I could do something that made me feel confident, which is something I lacked. I could also obtain a degree in the process.

After that, I figured I would be set for the rest of my life. I was taking baby steps towards college. I was afraid of getting ahead of myself. Occasionally, a fleeting, "*What if I'm not cut out for college*?" thought entered my mind. Those were the things that kept me up at night. I'd remind myself that I wasn't cut out for walking either, but I did that. I was told I wasn't cut out for mainstream classes, but I did those too.

According to the doctors from childhood, I wasn't even cut out to survive past my 10th birthday. I was a decade beyond my "expiration date." I hated relying on all the things I'd "overcome" to silence self-doubt, but at times, it was necessary. I truly didn't give myself enough credit for the way I did overcome so many challenges. I didn't know life without my challenges so all the "overcoming" I was doing just felt *normal.* I couldn't give myself credit for *normal* accomplishments.

After Nana's passing, dad inherited some money. It wasn't enough to make us wealthy, but it was just enough to get us out of the motel we'd lived in for the entire time I was in high school. Eleven months after spending my high school graduation night eating Big Mac meals in a poorly lit motel room, we finally moved into a modest three-bedroom home in a small Long Island suburb. It was only 30 minutes away from Mount Sinai, but eons away from that level of privilege. Aside from much-needed space, that house gave me something else. It gave me a place to go home to.

I knew if I went away to school, I could always come home. Also, I didn't feel as compelled to flee. When all I had to come "home" to every night was four people cramped in a single room with really bad decor, it left a lot to be desired. At that time, living in a dorm room with one other girl and eating ramen noodles for breakfast, lunch, and dinner actually sounded appealing. That was the biggest reason I wanted to go away. I wanted to be somewhere instead of living nowhere. Suddenly, things were comfortable. I had my own room, home-cooked meals since I wasn't living off whatever fast food my parents could find close to the motel anymore, and mom washed all our clothes. I was comfortable. Often comfort lends itself to complacency. I was no longer yearning to go away to college. I was becoming content with the thought of going to a local college and living at home.

With all this newfound space, Ashley and I drifted. We lived a room away but felt as if we were miles apart. As we both got older, we just couldn't find common ground. At its crux, there were feelings of jealousy and resentment that neither of us dared to speak of. Instead of seeing our commonalities, we viewed each other as vastly different. We each thought the other had things easier. When I saw Ashley, I saw a chubby girl whose only problem was that she needed to drop some weight. She was completely free from any disability. Nobody judged her intelligence based on the size of her waistline. I downplayed the fact that she was teased mercilessly. Sure, kids are mean. I was teased when I was her age. But I thought *at least the world won't be mean to her.* I loved my sister, but I hated the freedom she had to just *be*. When people mentioned her, she wasn't *Deborah and Lamont's fat daughter.* During all conversations that mentioned me, I was their *disabled daughter.*

Occasionally, someone familiar with disabilities would understand that I was a person first. They'd say *Deborah and Lamont's daughter in a wheelchair.* Ashley looked at me and saw the opposite. She saw my size zero frame. Thanks to the notorious Calvin Klein ads in the '90s, that was the ideal size. She was seemingly oblivious to the fact that I was only three feet tall. I wasn't going to grow much taller. When I got good grades, she thought that came easy. I didn't broadcast my struggles nearly as often as I touted my successes, so how could she know that A's didn't just fall in my lap? I wanted her to think that my grades were effortless. I wanted her to look up to me. She knew how hard things were for me physically, but she was still my baby sister. I wanted her to admire me.

Whatever the core reasons were, we'd come a long way from the two little girls who couldn't be without each other for more than a few minutes. Our relationship was a complex one. It wasn't until I was an adult that I learned we bonded over trauma. It was my trauma as much as it was hers. If I was in pain, she hurt too. When I had surgery and mom was with me, she had to stay with family. If I broke a bone and couldn't go in the pool, mom wouldn't let her go either, out of fairness. We had shared experiences that created extremely different reactions and altered our realities. Neither of us took the time to honor the other's reality. Instead, we villainized the other for not thinking, feeling, and living like the other did. It was unfair and nearly destroyed our relationship forever.

On a very conscious level, I desperately wanted to go to college. I dreamed of degrees, parties, sororities, and friendships that would last a lifetime — a college experience straight out of the movies. Subconsciously, though, I still heard the voices of the elementary school band teacher, Mr. Walters, the high school science teacher, and every other person who gave up on me before they even gave me a chance. I heard the resounding voice of doubt in my own head for what felt like decades.

The struggle was how could I believe in myself when no one else believed in me?

How could I move in the direction of success when people who are responsible for educating and setting me up for success instead spent nine years telling me that my failure was inevitable?

The answer was much simpler than I made it out to be. I didn't have to believe in myself. I just couldn't believe in them. The naysayers couldn't live rent-free in my head anymore. I was going to propel myself toward success because I was told that I couldn't. I was going to be successful because I was disabled, not *in spite* of it. I was going to college, not because I believed I could, but because people said I couldn't.

I spent most of my life believing the goal was to prove people wrong. What a waste of energy. I knew what I could do. I could feel my confidence growing. I just needed to prove *myself* right. By default, everyone who said can't, won't, or don't, should be wrong. That was a much needed mental shift. I knew the rest would fall into place. A weight lifted the minute I stopped trying to prove other people wrong and instead set out to prove myself right. I knew what I was capable of. I wasn't here to change the perceptions of who I was or what I could do. Perception is reality. How someone perceived me did not have to be my reality.

This Is College?

Five Towns College is a small private college in Suffolk County on Long Island. It wasn't just the student population that made them small. The building itself was a former middle school situated right off a busy highway. It may have been repurposed to be a college but never upgraded to look like a college. They liked to call themselves a "premier college for performing arts." Yet, the theater still looked like it was designed to hold a sixth-grade production of *Hello Dolly.* They were not NYU Tisch School of the Arts and I knew that. That didn't stop them from trying to sell it like it was. They offered me admission. As a 20-year-old coming out of a two-year gap year who still didn't fully believe I could get into college, admission was the most I thought I could ask for. The goal was to just go to college, right? Get a degree. It didn't matter from where. So Five Towns College it was. A four-year commitment to take classes at an overpriced "middle school." There wasn't a college savings account for me. Growing up, my parents barely made ends meet. Saving for me to go to college was not a priority. Yet, there was no shortage of loans and credit cards being offered. That made college appear affordable. In reality, all it did was make it attainable.

I never toured the college. I was there exactly one time before classes started and it was for my theater department audition, which was in the auditorium on the main level. It wasn't until my first day of classes that I learned the school was multiple floors and had no elevator. I expected the theater to be inaccessible. Most theaters are designed with stadium seating and stairs leading to and from the stage. I anticipated having to navigate a few stairs during my theater classes. However, I was fully unprepared for the entire school to be inaccessible. I thought I was protected from places like this. The ADA — which guaranteed that disabled people had equal access to public spaces — was signed into law 10 years earlier. *How did this school not have an elevator? Was equal subjective?*

I had watched my mom advocate for me for years. She would quickly confront business owners and managers the minute we encountered a place that was not accessible. Her favorite phrase was, "You are in violation of the ADA." I swear she knew that law better than the politicians who wrote it. I knew how to advocate for myself but rarely had to. I didn't have much of a social life in high school. I'd go to a friend's house once in a while. I knew the ADA didn't apply to homes. I didn't know many disabled people, so I was never shocked to see a flight of stairs in someone's home. But I wasn't in someone's home. I was in college. *My* college. I deserved access to the entire building.

My English class was on the lowest level. On my first day, I had no idea how I could get down there. I thought maybe this building had a secret elevator, so I went to the Dean's office for direction. David Cohen was the Dean. His father, Stanley, was the school's president. The only difference between the two was that Stanley doesn't meet with anyone. David confirmed there was no elevator.

"If you just take the path around the back of the building and enter the back door, you'll be on the lower level." That was the answer I got.

That was the first time I felt unseen. I felt so insignificant. It was easier to ignore my existence in this space rather than value me enough to make it possible for me to exist here.

The path that lead to the back door was narrow and eerie. This was long before rape culture was a rampant problem on college campuses, so safety was of little concern. My wheelchair barely fit entirely on the pavement. I often felt one of the wheels drift on the grass. In the fall and winter, that path was covered with leaves, snow, and ice that they didn't care enough to clear. I was supposed to be able to enter that back door but it was always locked. I'd pull on the handle, bang on the glass, and scream until someone finally let me in. It was degrading waiting outside for someone to let me into a place I should have never been locked out of in the first place.

Theater kids are sometimes the easiest kids to meet. They're willing to talk to anyone. They have little to no fear of being rejected. They spend their lives being rejected by directors and production companies. I quickly made friends with other theater students. We took all the same classes. We were a small tight-knit group of kids mostly from the Tri-State area. We were all a bit quirky, super outgoing, and we were all theater majors so there were no wallflowers among us. It was so much different than my high school experience. For the first time ever, I wasn't segregated. I was a part of the group. We took all the same classes. For the first time, I was the same as my peers. There were no lower expectations for me. There were no special education classes I could be forced into. Stage movement and dance were in the curriculum. I had to take them. I wanted to take them. The only time I felt different was when it was time to go to class. My friends would walk together and I would head to my designated path. It was the one thing that made me feel separated; missing out on the jokes and gossip often told in the hallways.

I never complained about it. It felt like a petty issue. Something that was too small to be upset about. Maybe I wasn't good at hiding how it made me feel because one by one they took turns carrying my wheelchair up and down the stairs. They never made me feel bad about it. It was just an act of simple kindness, but it meant the world to me. The action said *you're one of us.* I knew that they would have my back. They made me feel *seen.* I would have left that school if they were not there. It wasn't just that it was inaccessible. It was the idea that school officials had no plans to change the layout to accommodate wheelchair accessibility.

In addition to finding some great friends, I found professors who believed in me. Luke ran the theater department. He was the only director. He was pretty eccentric but extremely funny. He was the first person to call me talented. This school may not have been everything I wanted, but it was everything God knew I needed. I needed a place where I could learn to believe in myself again. It was also a place where I could truly test my physical limitations. I knew I could walk short distances and manage a few steps. I wasn't pushing past that. I quit physical therapy in high school. I didn't have the time. Between excessive studying and all my extracurricular activities, I was incredibly busy after school. Not to mention that because I was homeless, it was better to involve fewer adults in my life. So mom didn't protest too much when I told her I was done with physical therapy. I always viewed the goal as walking. I achieved that. As far as I was concerned, there was no need to continue. I didn't factor in all the things I should continue to improve. Conditioning, stamina, balance, and gait were lifelong improvements that were a natural progression for people who walk every day. For people who don't walk, these things must be practiced.

Part of the theater program was a musical theater dance class. I knew they were going to tell me I couldn't take it. I wasn't sure what they'd make me replace it with since it was part of my degree program. I was resolved not to be told what I could and couldn't do in college. I practiced all my rebuttals in my bedroom mirror to make sure my face looked stern enough if I had to fight to be allowed to take a class.

"I'm paying for these classes! So technically, you and every professor in that department work for me," I practiced.

Much to my surprise, I got no pushback from the administration when I added theatrical dance to my first semester schedule. Honestly, what could they have said? They were wholly unprepared for a disabled student. I knew that. They had no idea how to change or alter the program to accommodate a disabled theater major. That worked to my benefit because it kept them out of my way. They couldn't stop me from taking any class because they had no alternatives. They also couldn't keep me out of the theater program because that would be blatant discrimination. I probably had the most leverage and control over my education than I had ever had.

That dance class was brutal! I knew it would be challenging, but I greatly underestimated how challenging it actually was. I came in with no dance training. I had only been walking unaided for two years, and suddenly I was in this dance class doing a Bob Fosse dance routine. I would catch a glimpse of myself in the dance mirror and try not to visibly cringe. I hated full-length mirrors. I wasn't yet comfortable with how different my body looked. Spending most of my time in a wheelchair, I never noticed how my body measured up in comparison to my counterparts. I was a Little Person. I knew what that meant. I didn't know what it looked like for me. Looking at my reflection, I saw all the bones that were bowed — a common feature of people with OI. It may have been common, but it looked foreign to me because I never viewed my body upright. I saw a spine that could not hold me upright. I saw freakishly long arms paired with really short legs. I watched as I moved alongside everybody, desperately trying to keep up and pretending I was graceful. I would watch as the sweat would bead on my forehead. I loved seeing myself sweat. That was the physical manifestation of pushing beyond my limitations. After puberty, my fracture rate plateaued. That is just the nature of the disease. Once a person gets through puberty, the bones don't fracture as easily. I was not cured, although I acted like it. I hadn't broken anything since high school. I was never afraid to fracture something, and now the risk of fracturing something was greatly diminished. With the increased bone density, I was even more fearless. I knew I was forcing my body to do something that my genetics said I shouldn't be able to do. That was liberating. Before dance class, the only choreography I ever did was cross from stage right to stage left during a group chorus number in high school productions. Suddenly I was really dancing.

By my second year, there were major staff changes in the theater department. A "changing of the guard" of sorts. Jack Allison, a professional director who was a professor at NYU, was coming to Five Towns College as the new Chair of the theater department. I didn't want him to come. We had created this perfect little family. Myself, my theater class, and the current head of the theater department, Luke, were in this insulated bubble. We did shows together, took classes together, and I enjoyed this very inclusive secular environment we were in. I didn't want someone new coming in and disrupting that. I didn't want to *prove* myself to someone new. I didn't want to beg for acceptance. I didn't want to fall back into the headspace of doubting myself again. I was terrified that that was exactly what would happen.

All my fears were for nothing. Jack came in and ended up being the person who believed in me more than I ever believed in myself, second only to my mom. When I had every reason to doubt myself, Jack would find every reason plus one as to why I shouldn't. We worked closely together. I was his teacher's assistant. I managed his grade book, printed tests, and whatever other administrative task he threw at me. He invited me to be his assistant director on multiple productions. My greatest memories were when he let me be his assistant director on shows. I learned more about theater and life in general from that man. A late dinner after a long rehearsal coupled with a few glasses of wine would have Jack turn into some great philosopher. He was so worldly. He was the ultimate paradox and he loved that. He was an older Catholic man who mocked the stereotype of an old Catholic man from New Jersey. He seemed to have a joke for every occasion and was not one for political correctness. He was a grandfatherly figure with a warm hug for everybody. He also was unafraid to drop an F-bomb. Jack expected a lot, but he also gave a lot. When we had a show to put on, we knew we had to bring our very best. There was no negotiating. Your work ethic had to match Jack's or else don't show up. The extent of his gratitude and encouragement made it all worth it. He was incredibly creative and talented when he directed a show. To this day, he is still one of the most brilliant minds to cross my path.

I spent four years at Five Towns College and never got my damn elevator. I'll never understand why. It didn't sound that hard. It was not a major structural change. I wish my 20-year-old self had the courage to stand up for herself. I wish she had of made it a point to tell the Dean that the setup was unacceptable in a post-ADA world. I wish she told him that her $12,000 a year in tuition made her worthy of an elevator! Simply, I wish I had the courage to tell him I would take my money elsewhere. In reality, I didn't believe there was an elsewhere. That wasn't an option yet. I still only had a Special Ed high school education. Maybe after a year or two of stellar college grades I could transfer to UCLA. Maybe eventually they'd accept me. If I applied myself and *put my mind to it,* someday I'd be good enough for a *real school*. Five Towns wasn't my first choice. It probably never should have been a choice at all, but it's where I ended up. It wasn't perfect. I went for the degree and ended up staying for the people.

Please Choose Me

I met Ryan during my sophomore year of college. He transferred to Five Towns as a theater major. I was immediately enamored by him. He had spent time overseas studying theater. He was talented, witty, and smart. He was the quintessential SOHO artsy actor and musician who every nerdy theater girl dreams of meeting — scruffy good looks, long hair, and raw, unvarnished talent. He was just moody and aloof enough to feel like the "bad boy," yet polite and respectful enough that my mom liked him. I didn't know it then but he'd be my first heartbreak. It wouldn't be the star-crossed lovers' heartbreak that I saw in the movies. I unintentionally broke my own heart.

I didn't date in high school. I was never asked out. I was the girl who got stood up for prom. I envied the girls who had boyfriends. I'd watch them walk through the halls holding hands. I wanted that, but in high school, it didn't seem attainable. I wasn't the pretty girl. I never saw anyone who looked like me in movies, magazines, or on television. On the few occasions I did see a disabled woman, she was not walking hand-in-hand with a man. Representation matters. Because I never saw disabled love, I just assumed that was something I couldn't have. It felt aspirational, but unrealistic. Mom never pushed me to date, but I know she wished I would have gone out more. She would tell me, "Mr. Right is not just going to show up at our front door."

Love wasn't on my radar until I met Ryan. I had a few hookups with guys I'd meet online. One carefully crafted dating profile after the next. I looked great on paper because I left out all the things I felt made me unappealing to men. According to my profile, I was "petite," and I told people, "I can't walk long distances." I wasn't lying. These were half-truths. To me, it sounded slightly better than, "I'm a Little Person who spent most of her life in a wheelchair." Some of the men who did know I was a Little Person fetishized the idea of me. I knew most, if not all, of these guys I'd never see again. I hated that most of these encounters lacked any real substance. It was fun, and gave me a quick confidence boost but I knew I wasn't on track to finding "the one." I hadn't connected with anyone before Ryan. I felt an almost immediate connection to him, or rather, I misinterpreted it as a connection. It was more a codependency than anything. I needed to be validated and made to feel important. He wanted the same. Ryan sought acceptance and to feel understood. Was I looking for a boyfriend or a project? Probably a little of both. He was the closest thing I knew to being in love. I didn't even know what it meant to be in love with myself. I had no business dating anyone. God had put my love life on pause for a reason. I paid no attention to the fact that I didn't yet have the capacity to love myself. Another person couldn't heal me, but I was willing to try and heal someone else.

Ryan and I became fast friends. Our friendship blossomed and we became super close. In what felt like minutes, I was head over heels in love with him. In reality, we only had an insanely codependent and ambiguous friendship. There were no clear boundaries, besides the fact that he was having sex with everyone else except me. I was constantly pouring into his cup, hoping that he'd give me the smallest modicum of validation. I lived for moments when he would say, "Hey, beautiful!" or compliment me in any way. I don't know if it was intentional on his part, but he gave me just enough attention to keep me hanging on his every word, but not enough that I'd think he wanted a future with me. It didn't matter because I wanted a future with him.

As if I wasn't falling for Ryan fast enough, Jack put me "in charge" of him. Ryan wasn't always the most likable person in the theater department. Ryan butted heads with Jack once in a while, but it was undeniable that he was talented. He was always the top contender for the male lead in our shows. Jack did not want to lose him to another school, and he needed other actors to be willing to work with him. Jack didn't expect me to make him likable, but told me, "He likes you more than he likes anyone else in this damn department." I knew that if that statement was true, it meant he was choosing me.

Our 12-hour days between classes and rehearsal started to include a lot of personal time. We spent hours practicing lines, watching movies, doing homework, and just being together. I let myself give in to the fantasy of him. We had inside jokes, he wrote me songs, we sang duets. It was every cliche you can think of when it comes to "theater people" dating. I was swept up in the idea of that same cliche. I was ready to just fast-forward through college, and get to this romanticized version of a future with him. The ambiguity of our relationship left me feeling like I was already his girlfriend. He was what I had been waiting for. I saw my children in his eyes. I saw this blissful life with my actor husband, where we both worked on Broadway, ate sushi, and read plays to each other late into the night.

I pursued him with everything I had. When he was feeling down, I made sure I was the one to build him up. He was super emotional and sensitive. I knew and used every opportunity to calm his emotional storm. I thought that if I always gave him what he needed, he would have no choice but to see me as wife material. If he saw how nurturing and loving I could be towards him, clearly he'd know what a great mother and wife I could be. I felt the resistance on his end. I wasn't sure what was causing it. Or maybe I did know but didn't want to admit it. I held onto everything that made me feel good and ignored everything that made me feel like crap. I tried not to pay attention when he talked about his most recent sexual escapade. Often they were with girls that I knew. I'd pout and pretend to be angry, but I always let it go. I rationalized that *half* of someone's love was better than none at all.

He *did* love me, though. I remember the first time he said it. It was my birthday and we were in my backyard. We had both been drinking. I don't know if it was the alcohol but he bent down in front of me and said, "I love you." My heart jumped right out of my chest. I thought, *tell the boy or he'll think you're not interested.*

"I love you too! I have loved you, but I thought it was too soon to say it," I said.

"You can say it anytime."

He bent down and kissed me. I expected to feel like some magical kiss out of a Disney movie. It wasn't. The minute our lips touched, I opened my eyes.

Is this really happening?

Then, nothing happened. This was a kiss like the one you gave your grandmother. I didn't realize that until I was moving my tongue and only feeling my own teeth. *Oh, it's one of* those *kisses.* I'm almost surprised I didn't say it out loud. I wanted him to love me like I loved him, but it wasn't the same.

He did love me, but he didn't *love* me.

A Real-Life Dwarf

Ask any actor and they'll tell you they just want to act, regardless of the role. I was no different. I was rarely cast. Luke cast me in the Thornton Wilder play *The Skin Of Our Teeth* during freshman year. I got to play Esmerelda, a fortune teller. It was a small role, but I was grateful. After all, I was only a freshman. I shouldn't have been expecting anything, but I had dreams of meaty roles. I wanted to be Abigail in *The Crucible*, Martha in *Who's Afraid of Virginia Wolf*, and Catherine in *The Heiress*. The problem was that I didn't fit any of those roles. Colorblind-style casting is great in theory but never seems to apply to disabled actors.

By definition, I have dwarfism. I am a real-life dwarf. Outside of Snow White and the Seven Dwarves, there were no roles written for people who looked like me. I knew my options as an actress would be limited. I learned in college that these roles were non-existent. I had the urge to rage against that, but I also was being taught the history of great American plays and musicals. In the time of Arthur Miller and Edward Albee, people who looked like me were left alone in institutions to rot. Little people with disabilities were not even on the radar of these playwrights as existing. Logically, I understood that most art is inspired by lived experiences and societal norms. What I couldn't reconcile is how a playwright could imagine witches, fortune tellers, and sorcerers but never imagined someone disabled.

Seemingly out of thin air, Jack and the musical director invented the Children's Theater program. I can't say they created it *for* me, but they knew they'd find me roles in children's shows. They didn't know how to fit me in traditional shows, but they knew that I was an acting major, and fulfilling the requirements of my degree meant I needed to act.

Our inaugural season of Children's Theater opened with a production of *Rumpelstiltskin*. I remember when Jack told me that I was cast as the main character. He'd asked if I'd seen the cast list and said, "You're the lead!"

It's Rumpelstiltskin! Not exactly the depth I was hoping for. I was grateful to have a chance to be on stage. Like any actor, I wanted to work. The question was, at what cost?

I was always cast as a troll or some other woodland creature. After all, not much exists in shows written for kindergarten children. As if it wasn't bad enough that my theater career was disappearing and looking more like a Dr. Seuss book, I was asked to do some really demeaning things. My blocking always included jumping up and down to get something out of reach, climbing, or some other action that drew attention to my height for laughs. I was relegated to a caricature of a Little Person. I still, to this day, don't know why I participated in that. Why didn't I stand up and say, "This is not okay?" I would have never participated in any Minstrel Show or sideshow-type buffoonery. This was no different. At the time, I didn't feel like I had the right to say anything because actors take direction.

Phil, who headed the Children's Theater program and directed the shows, was insensitive at best. To try and explain that I was feeling demeaned seemed like a fruitless effort. I also knew if not for these roles, I would not be on stage at all. I was still struggling to find my voice too. I didn't want to rock the boat or bite the hand that fed me. So, I allowed myself and my disability to be exploited for laughs. No one made me do anything, but everyone capitalized on the fact that I just wanted to work.

I regret those shows. All of them. It's not an excuse but I was so damn naive. I didn't pay attention to the fact that I was standing on the shoulder of giants. So many disabled people came before me and fought for my right to just live equitably. I was willfully ignoring that legacy and perpetuating grossly inaccurate stereotypes. I wish I could redo those days. It was so much bigger than me and my acting career. As a disabled woman, as a Little Person, I had a responsibility to advance the progress and conversation surrounding those communities, not mock it.

My Head Is Killing Me

I was a junior on course to graduate with a Bachelor of Fine Arts. I was an honors student with straight As. If I kept my current pace, I was most likely going to graduate Magna Cum Laude. That was once something I only dreamed of, and suddenly it was within reach. I was an integral part of the theater department, still working one-on-one with Jack. We had multiple shows in production and I was working on all of them. I was easily the happiest I had ever been. I was busy and I always did best when I was juggling multiple things. I thrived under pressure. That is probably why I took on more than I should have. Because I knew my best work was born out of external pressure.

Seemingly out of nowhere, I started getting these awful headaches. The first time I felt one was when I headed into rehearsal for a children's show that I was in. I felt this piercing pain deep in my brain. The feeling stunned me and I winced. One of the other cast members asked if I was okay.

"Yeah, my head is killing me," I responded.

She asked me when I had last eaten. I skipped breakfast that morning so that was probably the source of the pain. I attributed the sudden pain to low blood sugar and went to rehearsal.

Only the pain didn't subside, even after I ate lunch. It persisted that day and well into the next. It increased in intensity, moving from one localized spot deep in my brain to encompassing my whole head. There was nothing that made the pain better, but everything made it worse. The bright white halogen lighting in the school was excruciating. The sound of my own chewing was like a buzz saw going off inside my head, not that I was eating much because I was so nauseous. Even the smell of food made me want to throw up. Garlic was the worst. Painkillers gave no relief. I would take three ibuprofen and chase those with two Aleve every few hours, and was still in pain. I tried everything people told me. I was living off Coca-Cola because someone mentioned the benefits of caffeine and it was the only thing that didn't make me want to throw up. I was constantly squeezing the fleshy spot between my thumb and index finger because someone told me that touching those pressure points relieved headaches. I always had a friend willing to rub my head and provide the scalp massages that should have offered relief. I'd even sprawl on the couch for hours with a cold washcloth draped across my eyes because cooling my eyelids was supposed to help relieve headaches. Nothing gave me relief. The pain was so bad that on nights when I was lucky enough to fall asleep, I would wake in more pain than I was when I drifted off to sleep.

Finally, the pain became so unbearable mom forced me to go to the emergency room. I had been reluctant to go because I didn't want to miss class, and I had to attend rehearsal every night. There just weren't enough hours in my day to squeeze in being sick. It had been years since I'd been in an emergency room. I hadn't broken anything since high school so there hadn't been a need.

The emergency room hadn't changed much. The walls were still institutional white and it smelled like a strange mix of bleach and vomit. The intake nurse asked why I was there as she took my vitals. I thought I had already told her. Maybe I hadn't. I really couldn't remember much. The days just seemed to all blend together.

"My head is killing me!" I said.

"Well, what does it feel like?" she asked.

I stared at her blankly trying to comprehend that question. *What does it feel like?* It was like nothing I had ever experienced before, and I was no stranger to pain.

"It's the worst headache of my life!" I blurted out.

The nurse left and I sat there trying to keep my eyes closed to keep out the light. *Why are hospital lights so bright?* The doctor walked in. He was in his mid-30s and wore a stark white lab coat.

"I hear you have a migraine." His high-pitched voice reverberated through my skull.

"It's not a migraine. I don't get migraines!" I snapped. At most, I got a headache every once in a while. I had no experience with migraines, but it sounded too normal to explain what I was feeling.

"Well, perhaps this is your first. Migraines are quite common." Something about the way he said that let me know he wasn't taking me seriously.

"No. Something is wrong. My head is killing me and has been for days!" I said, almost pleading.

"We'll get a CAT scan and have a look," he said, most likely only to appease me.

In less than an hour, I had the CAT scan done and the doctor had the results.

"There's nothing there!" he said boastfully. An emergency room doctor, not a neurologist, declared me fine and ready to send me home. I spent more time in the waiting room than I did being examined.

"You should get a specialist," I said.

"The images don't lie. It's just a really bad headache," he said. I wasn't expecting him to find a tumor, but something was wrong and I knew it.

"You're a college student, right?" he asked.

"Yes," I said through gritted teeth.

"It's midterm time. You're probably up late studying and stressed out. These look like stress headaches to me."

What the hell does he mean they look like stress headaches?

I didn't know if this guy was just a jerk or severely underqualified. Perhaps he was a little bit of both. I left the emergency room in just as much pain as I arrived in and with absolutely no answers.

Mom and I would make several more trips to the ER over the next eight weeks. Every time I was met with some doctor who thought I was exaggerating my level of pain and another CAT scan or MRI that showed nothing. Whatever that first doctor wrote in my chart haunted me because every time I was seen, I was diagnosed as an over-achiever suffering from stress headaches. You're damn right I was an over-achiever. I had to be because I learned early that I had to outwork my peers because people wanted to give up on the girl in the wheelchair. But people aren't as quick to give up on the hard workers or the determined. But I knew my work ethic and determination were not the cause of my headaches. On my last trip to the ER, the attending physician suggested I see a psychiatrist instead of continuing to come to the ER. Again, they said that the source of my headaches was stress and possible anxiety that I was not aware of.

I felt hopeless. I was in debilitating pain. I couldn't eat. I couldn't sleep. I was being told that maybe I was feeling all these symptoms simply because I was crazy. I may have briefly even questioned my own sanity. I was stressed and under a lot of pressure but I always thrived under pressure. It wasn't something that was suddenly going to make me lose my mind. In order to take mental illness off the table, I started seeing a psychiatrist. He was a nice guy. He offered me some water before I sat down. It quickly became clear that he had no interest in hearing why I was there. He prescribed me Prozac for depression. I didn't get the memo that I had depression. He gave me Ambien to sleep and to top off this medication cocktail, he added Xanax for good measure. He was treating perceived emotional pain while I was exhibiting physical symptoms.

My family was almost as frustrated as they were concerned. I turned off the lights in every room in the house. We were living in darkness and it still wasn't dark enough to lessen the pain in my head. Despite mom making complete meals, I could not eat. The physical act of chewing felt like my skull was literally splitting in two. I'd try to stick to the soft foods. Mom was always willing to make me some instant mashed potatoes or canned soup. Anything that wasn't liquid sent me running to the bathroom to throw up. I was tired of throwing up. My throat was raw and my breath stunk. It was just easier not to eat.

I was getting used to feeling hungry. I was living off of Coca-Cola and coffee that I'd get at school. I lost 20 pounds. I was on Prozac, but still depressed. I didn't even know what I was sad about. The only thing that kept me from crying is that the act of sobbing wreaked havoc on my head. I was taking Ambien but still not sleeping. Maybe that was because of all the coffee I was drinking. I would drag myself to school every day and to rehearsal all night. If I wasn't sleeping anyway, might as well do something productive with the time. I was physically weak. I struggled to shower in the dark because turning the lights on was not an option. I was so tired of people pointing out that I "look exhausted" or telling me to "get some sleep." I would if I could. On the rare night when I did fall asleep, I'd wake up with my heart racing and my head throbbing.

The psychiatric drugs numbed everything else but the pain in my head. I had moments when I couldn't feel my left hand. Then, I'd lose feeling in my whole arm. Eventually, the feeling would return. I wished my head would go numb. I just did not want to feel this level of pain anymore. It was worse than any broken bone I ever had. I had no thoughts other than the pain. I don't know how I kept it together as well as I did. I was physically, emotionally, and mentally drained.

Thursday, April 3, 2003, was a mild early spring night. It was also the night that nearly derailed my entire life. We were in rehearsal for the Cole Porter musical *Anything Goes*. There was a costume parade on schedule, so the costume designer could see the cast in full costume. As assistant director, I went to all scheduled rehearsals. I wanted to be everywhere Jack was. I hoped to soak up all his knowledge. Even he skipped the rehearsals dedicated to costumes, though. I knew that it wasn't vital for me to attend. Our costume designer was very nice, but she was also very loud and unorganized. As she screamed for our lead actor, I just knew that I wasn't going to be able to tolerate her energy based on how I was feeling.

"Tim, try these pants!" she bellowed out.

I went to my stage manager, Niki, and asked if I could leave.

"My head is killing me," I explained.

That phrase had become commonplace between all my friends and me.

I knew rehearsal could go on without me. I needed to lie down. I felt guilty asking to leave even though I knew Niki didn't need me. Niki had been a stage manager for much bigger productions than this one.

I wasn't asking permission. Subconsciously, I was putting someone on notice. I was telegraphing that if I didn't return, they should come looking for me. I knew something was gravely wrong. This was more than just a headache. I started feeling very sleepy and confused. There were mats in the gym. I thought if I could just take a quick nap, I could return to rehearsal feeling better. I still felt compelled to tell someone where I was. I knew I could trust Niki. They weren't an alarmist. Instead, they were very practical and pragmatic. Out of everyone I knew, Niki would notice if I didn't come back but wouldn't panic the entire cast. I clumsily walked up the theater stairs and stumbled into the hallway.

Where is the gym?

I'm not even sure I knew what a gym was anymore. I stumbled through the halls with my eyes barely open. The hallway lights were too bright. It was as if all of my senses were amplified to an unbearable level. I never found the gym but passed our dance studio. It looked vaguely familiar. I had classes in there. I spent hours rehearsing in there. Jack's office was down there. This was a place I knew. I gripped the railing and navigated down the three steps. I walked into the studio and saw the mats I had been looking for. I collapsed onto one.

I fell asleep. I rolled onto my back, staring blankly into the ceiling light. I noticed that something was different. The lights didn't feel like lasers burning my brain anymore. The minute I realized that, the whole room went black. Finally, I was in complete darkness. This was the darkness I'd been seeking for 8 weeks. I had enough consciousness to realize the room seemed completely black but not enough consciousness to know the room was still lit.

I had just lost my sense of sight.

There was just a sense of nothingness. I saw nothing. I heard nothing. I felt nothing. I didn't even feel my head anymore.

Finally, there was something. There was sound. Niki and my friend Vanessa entered. I could hear them calling my name, but I struggled to see them. They asked me questions that I couldn't answer. I struggled to identify the voices but I couldn't understand any of the words being spoken. It was like listening to a poorly tuned radio — everything was garbled. I thought, *I need help.* For the first time, I felt something. I felt fear. I needed them to know I was not just asleep.

Then, I saw something. It was Vanessa's long red hair, but I couldn't make out shapes or see with any clarity. There was no mistaking the cascade of red hair falling on my face as she looked at me.

"Who should we call?" Vanessa asked frantically. That question was probably for Niki and not me.

"Mom," I said as I drooled from the left side of my mouth.

Vanessa's immediate follow-up question was, "What's her phone number?"

I didn't remember her phone number in that moment. I barely remembered Vanessa even though she was standing right in front of me.

"Cell phone!" is the last thing I remember hearing. Finally, a voice I recognized. It was Niki. The fear subsided. During my last moment of consciousness, I thought, *Niki knew to find me! Niki and Vanessa are here. I'm not alone.* I then went completely unconscious.

There's no way they could have known it then, and they wouldn't learn it for almost two weeks, but they saved my life that night.

By the time my parents arrived, I had lost control of my bladder and bowel and was lying in my own vomit. Mom said that half of my body felt like I had a fever and the other side was ice cold. Out of fear and in the absence of all rational behavior, my parents decided not to call an ambulance but to drive me to a hospital 45 minutes away. Mom had an affinity for Stony Brook Hospital. It was the hospital that took such great care of me as a child. It was also the hospital that sent me home several times with a diagnosis of "stress headaches" for the past eight weeks. For whatever reason, she wanted me there. Dad obliged. I was totally unconscious. The two of them got me into Jack's office chair, which they carefully carried up a small flight of stairs, and pushed me out to mom's Ford Explorer.

Dad drove 80 miles an hour on the Long Island Expressway where the max speed limit is 65. Dad loves to tell this story. He took a Suffolk County Police officer on a high-speed *chase* that ended at the hospital emergency room entrance, with the police officer drawing his gun on mom and dad. Dad tried to explain to the officer that I was in need of emergency medical attention, while mom frantically ran inside looking for help. Doctors came to the truck and immediately took my vitals. They confirmed for the officer that this was a medical emergency. I was alive, but barely. The officer offered his well wishes and left.

I was dying. My blood pressure was low, which is often a clear indication of bleeding. Yet, there was no visible blood. My heart rate had slowed, and I was unconscious. A series of imaging scans revealed I had a massive brain bleed — an intracerebral hemorrhage, or hemorrhagic stroke, in my right hemisphere. Simply put, the right side of my brain was drowning in my own blood and immediate intervention was needed. My chances at survival were slim.

The hospital called the on-call neurosurgeon since emergency rooms don't have neurosurgeons wandering the halls. Dr. Fredrick Guttman arrived and that was nothing short of divine intervention. I don't think I will ever not believe that he was sent by God that night because I wasn't supposed to die. Dr. Guttman spent eleven hours performing a full craniotomy. He removed a portion of my skull, allowing him access to the right side of my brain. He evacuated the pool of blood that filled my head and cauterized the bleeding vessel. My brain was swollen from the trauma. The skull bone was replaced and secured with metal screws. He drilled three holes in the remaining bone to allow for external tubes to drain any residual blood or cerebral spinal fluid. I was put into a medically induced coma. This was to allow my brain time to rest and for the swelling to reduce.

Mom recalled the heart-stopping moment that Dr. Guttman appeared in the doorway of the surgical waiting room. She breathlessly wanted him to tell her that I was okay. But that is not exactly what he said.

"She's okay for now. I did everything I could do. The rest is between her and God," he told mom.

Mom was strong in her faith and would later tell me that when Dr. Guttman invoked God's name, she knew it was okay. She took that as a sign that she could rest because God was in control. Mom was like that. Whenever she faced a situation where all control was taken from her, she would surrender and simply say, "Give it to God!"

I was alive, but that's all anyone knew. As I lay there blissfully unaware, there was no telling what the true extent of injury to my brain was. For 8 weeks, blood had been slowly dripping out of a blood vessel. It was only a slow leak until it ruptured. When the blood itself comes in contact with the brain tissue, it causes brain damage. It can cause sections of the brain to die.

Mom told me I was never alone. She, Alex, Ashley, and Dad were there. She said they'd trade off when one needed to eat, sleep, or go home. Mom had given Ryan updates on my condition. It wasn't long before the entire theater department knew I was in a coma. Jack told me that during that time, he would say a prayer for me before heading to rehearsal. I wish I could have felt all of the love and prayers. In retrospect, it might have been better that I couldn't because that would have meant that I would have felt all of their trepidation as we all wondered whether or not I would be able to speak, walk, or even move.

The bleed had originated in my right hippocampus, allowing blood to flow through the temporal lobe and into the parietal lobe before pooling between my temporal and occipital lobes on the same side. This meant that the biggest threats were to my memory and my eyesight. OI left me with poor eyesight to begin with. *Would I be blind now?* It was all so uncertain. I was glad I got to sleep through that part of it.

Five days later, they slowed the IV medication that kept me in the coma and allowed me to wake up. I opened my eyes and blinked several times. They didn't focus immediately. I wore contact lenses and was familiar with blurry vision, but this was different. I saw outlines and colors, but did not see them separately. One shape blended into the other. My head felt heavy. It almost felt too big for my body. Like that one time dad took me for a motorcycle ride, and I had to wear a helmet twice the size of my head. I felt the pressure of my very swollen head and some residual swelling of my brain.

I heard my stomach growl. Up until 8 weeks ago, I could out-eat grown men. Up until 8 weeks ago, a standard post-rehearsal dinner was 4 tacos from Taco Bell and a chalupa. I was hungry. Not hungry for coffee, but hungry for real food. I was confused. I could smell the distinct sterile, overly clean smell of bleach. *I was in a hospital.* But not a hospital waiting room because there wasn't the recent odor of old women wearing way too much perfume. I had no memory of the days leading up to my waking up. My throat and mouth were extremely dry. I tried calling out for my mom but I had a breathing tube down my throat. I wanted somebody to explain what had happened but nobody said anything. They all just stood there staring at me, like a zoo exhibit. I knew they were all just relieved to see me awake, moving and trying to communicate. While they were all breathing a collective sigh of relief, I was becoming more agitated, and God I was thirsty. I darted my eyes around, trying to make them focus.

Finally, they did focus and I saw them: those God-awful pink and mint-green drapes flanking the window. I gripped the sheets in panic. *I've been here before.* I was *in* the hospital. No one answered my questions because I couldn't ask questions. I noticed that right below my nose was a white loop. I wasn't 100% sure what it was but I could tell it was attached to the tube in my mouth. Ever since I was a kid, I've removed things that make me uncomfortable. In middle school, I had Ashley help me cut a cast off with an Exacto knife I took from art class. This tube was making me more uncomfortable than any cast I'd ever had. I hooked my index finger in that loop and pulled. Mom screamed. The doctor and nurse ran inside the room. I gagged. I choked. My throat was on fire. I extubated myself and I was breathing on my own.

"What happened?" I asked.

"We'll talk about it," mom said, as if not wanting to upset me.

I don't know what she thought she was hiding. I literally just pulled a breathing tube out of my throat. I knew something bad had happened.

"Mom? Please," I said, looking up at her.

My eyes focused on her face. I wanted to know what happened. I didn't remember anything, but I knew whatever happened was major.

"A week ago, you had a brain hemorrhage," she told me. "You're in the ICU. You've been in a coma for the past five days, but you're doing well, they say."

I could hear the concern in her voice. I was overcome with emotions and just started weeping. Mom held me. She held me tighter than she'd held me since I was a little girl.

The only thing I could remember immediately was the headaches. The pain had been so unbearable that I didn't think it was possible to forget it. Every emotion I felt was so visceral, and the very first one was anger. For 8 weeks I had been begging for help. I was saying something was wrong with my head and nobody believed me. *Now here I was in the ICU after spending five days in a coma?* I almost didn't have the capacity to process that. Doctors had told me I was crazy. They said I was stressed. They repeatedly sent me home. *How could people who do this for a living miss something as important as a bleeding brain?*

After two days of being out of the coma, the blank spots started to fill in my memories. School was at the forefront. I had tests to take and shows to put on. *Anything Goes* was set to open on April 26th. I had to be there. For my British Lit class, I had to read *Sir Gawain and the Green Knight*. I finished it the morning of the hemorrhage, and knew I had a test coming up but couldn't remember when and didn't even know what day it was. A nurse came in to check my wound and give me my meds. She seemed to know my medication schedule. Maybe she'd seen my class schedule, too.

"Excuse me, I have a test on a book I just read. Can you find out what day that is for me?" I asked.

"Baby girl, this is the hospital. You're not in school," she said in a thick Jamaican accent.

"Well, what day is it? I'm going back to school soon. As soon as I'm out of here," I told her.

"Baby girl, you need to rest and recover now. You can worry about school later." There was something comforting about her calling me baby girl, and her accent masked that she was dismissing my questions about school.

"But what day is today? I have a show that opens on the 26th. I need to be there for that."

She looked at me and smiled. She could tell I was not letting up. I needed the date.

"It's April 10th today. You get better and get home first. Then worry about school and whatever shows you have."

Clearly, this woman didn't know me. I was going to lie in that bed and obsess over school and all my shows until I was released from the hospital and got back to class.

I spent two weeks in the hospital. At that time, I tried to assess what my life looked like now. My memory felt fragmented. I couldn't feel the entire left side of my body, I had lost a significant portion of my peripheral vision, and I was unsteady on my feet. But those unforgiving headaches were gone. Doctors suggested I take the rest of the semester off. They recommended I take a medical leave of absence. That was not going to happen. I was finally a straight-A student. I was finally more than just the girl in a wheelchair. I was a director, a teacher's assistant, an actress, a friend, and "smart." I was not trading all that in to become the girl with the brain injury. For the first time in ten weeks, I was not in debilitating pain. I didn't stay home when I was in pain so there was no reason to do so now.

The day I arrived home was cathartic. I was so relieved to be pain-free, and I was excited to sleep in my own bed and eat meals with my family. It's so interesting how much I missed the little things, like eating with my family, the minute it was taken away. I was most excited to get back to school.

I was able to move around my house freely. There was no IV pole that I had to drag around with me or a well-meaning nurse demanding that I allow them to escort me to and from the bathroom. I had privacy for the first time in two weeks. I was still unsteady on my feet but I made my way down the hallway to the bathroom. The main bathroom, the one Ashley and I shared, had a wall that was a full mirror. As I entered, I saw my reflection staring back at me. I looked different than I remembered. I used this mirror every morning to put makeup on. This was the mirror that caused me to throw an eyeliner pencil at it in frustration because I could never get close enough to perfectly line my eyes on the first try. Today, I was almost too close. I looked up and in a moment and realized that my head had been shaved. The whole time I was in the hospital, my head was wrapped in bandages to protect the drains and incisions. Nobody prepared me for the fact that the entire right side of my head had been shaved. The left side was still the length I remembered it. I looked like I was about to star in the musical *Jekyll and Hyde*. I burst into tears.

I immediately felt horrible for being this upset over my hair. I felt ungrateful. I had just survived a near-death experience. By the grace of God, I was still alive, and on my first day home, I was sobbing over freaking hair. As soon as I composed myself, I apologized to God. I thanked God for sparing my life and apologized for being so upset over hair. I asked for forgiveness. Then, I went into my room and tried every possible version of a comb-over. I tried bandannas and headbands. I wanted anything to help salvage what was left of my hair. It wasn't just hair. It was my femininity. It was my style, and it had all been left on the floor of the operating room.

Mom came to my room and did what she always did so brilliantly: she consoled me and showed me a way to do what needed to be done.

"It'll grow back," she said.

I knew it would eventually grow back, but I looked like a hot mess. Ashley tried to remind me that mom gave me a mirror to see my head when I was in the hospital. I was on so many narcotics to control the pain during my hospital stay. I didn't remember that. And it didn't matter.

"Let's just shave the other side. It will all grow back together at the same speed," Mom suggested. "Besides, you can pull off short hair. You have a heart-shaped face and a small head. Now, your sister, on the other hand, can never go bald!"

We both laughed, and with that, she grabbed dad's clippers and shaved the rest of my head. As I watched the hair fall to the ground like dandelion seeds on a windy spring day, I felt lighter. I was devastated that my hair was gone, but I searched for things to be grateful for. My headaches were gone, and at 23 years old, I just cheated death. As I looked at myself in the mirror, I rubbed my head. I felt the holes that were left by the drains. I ran my finger along my 10-inch scar and thought, "*This is what it looks like to walk through hell and come out victorious.*" At that moment, I felt proud.

Against the advice of doctors, and much to the chagrin of my parents, I returned to school two days after being released from the hospital. Mom asked me to consider staying home for at least a week. That wasn't even a consideration I'd made, and she didn't fight me on it. I know she wanted to, but she resisted the urge. I promised her I'd call often and let her know that I was okay. I reminded her how loved and protected I was by Jack and the entire theater department. After all, if Niki and Vanessa hadn't looked for me, we wouldn't even be discussing me going back to school. I would be dead.

Ryan gave mom his word. He would drive me to and from school. He'd also walk me to my classes. It's interesting how almost dying can remind people of how much they care.

Anything Goes was set to open on April 26th. I had made a silent promise to my cast and crew that I'd be there. Come hell or high water, I was going to keep that promise. I didn't feel right just showing up to school at call time and not going to classes that day. I viewed my classes and my shows with the same regard. One wasn't more important than the other. They both required my effort and focus. I had been juggling a part-time job, a full-time class schedule, and multiple shows simultaneously for three years. There was no need to stop now. That day I walked through the front doors of Five Towns College the most fearless and confident I had ever been in my entire life. I truly believed that there was nothing I couldn't accomplish. Something about staring down death makes you feel like a superhero. The feeling, however, was short-lived.

I met Niki in the theater, script in hand and fully prepared to sit backstage. Jack stopped me.

"You're not going back there!" Jack shouted.

"She's good. She's just going to sit backstage. There's nothing she needs to do!"

I loved Niki for immediately coming to my defense. Niki knew I was not going to take being sidelined lightly. Jack looked at me for a minute. Sometimes, when Jack stared at me, it felt like he was trying to communicate with my soul.

"You don't need to be backstage! You're an audience member tonight," he told me.

I wanted to protest. I knew I didn't need to be backstage, but I wanted to be there. For 8 weeks, while my brain bled, I was backstage. I didn't miss a beat, but at that moment, I felt like now that the show was up, Jack was casting me aside. For the first time in our relationship I was truly mad at him. He had always been on my side, at times being my biggest cheerleader. Now, he had become one of the "can't" and "don't" people I encountered. I knew he was right, and I knew Jack cared deeply. It was frustrating because caring often leads to unnecessary worry. I always found myself on the receiving end of worry. I love that people care, but worry often quickly turns into smothering. I spent my whole life earning my right to be independent. When other people worry, my independence is threatened.

I took my script and sat in the front row of the theater. I was an audience member. I'd seen dozens of shows on Broadway. I know how to be an audience member: I sit, I silence my cell phone when the lights go down, I clap at the end of dance numbers, and I laugh at every corny joke. Audience members have no connection or investment in the production. The problem was that I didn't know how to be an audience member for shows I worked behind the scenes on. The show I was expected to passively watch had been my life for weeks. I coached actors, learned lighting cues, knew the blocking, and memorized every line. I was not some foot-tapping audience member who could just sit there, but I tried.

It wasn't just Jack. My family expected me to slow down. I knew I was still incredibly weak, but I wasn't going to recover at the pace I wanted by doing so much less, which felt like doing nothing. As a result of the surgery, the part of my brain that was affected made me an emotional wreck. I cried nearly every day. Recovery was extremely hard. What should have been a simple task like putting on my shoes felt like a perplexing puzzle. I wasn't particularly good at puzzles. When I was a kid, I pulled all the stickers off my Rubik's Cube and rearranged them so it looked like I solved it after trying to solve it too many times. For me, puzzles always felt like they weren't meant to be solved.

Putting shoes on should be simple. It's something I've been doing since I was little. All of a sudden, I couldn't put them on the right feet. Once they were on, they looked right. Maybe they felt a little awkward, but visually, they looked right. Mom or dad would point out that they were on the wrong feet. I would dissolve into a puddle of tears. On the rare occasions that I successfully put them on the right feet, I stared at the laces. My fingers felt foreign and I was admittedly unsure of how I wanted them to move. It reminded me of when I was learning to play the flute. I knew where the keys were but my fingers were unfamiliar with the configuration.

My memory felt fractured, but that was the only thing that seemed to be getting better. Every day I'd get more of my long-term memories back. They weren't cohesive storylines. They were more like jumbled images and random phrases, but I remembered being a child. I remembered what classes I was taking. I may not have remembered how to get to the classroom, but I knew what class it was. If it made it into my long-term memory, it was still in there. Slowly, the story of my life was piecing itself back together.

On one of my first days back, I was scheduled to go to my British literature class. It just so happened to be the day we were supposed to take the test on *Sir Gawain and the Green Knight.* I wasn't entirely confident about it, but I did read the book before my stroke. I never had a problem with reading comprehension or recalling what I'd read. My near-perfect memory is what got me through most tests. Dr.

Kelley, the professor, pulled me aside and urged me not to take the test. I had missed two weeks of school and all my professors had been told what had happened. I was put off by the suggestion that I shouldn't take the test. I hated every damn minute of that book, but I read it. I wanted to take the test and never think about that book again.

"I can take the test," I said.

"But you just got out of the hospital," he countered.

Logically, I knew Dr. Kelly meant no harm. He recognized the severity of what I had just gone through. Emotionally, though, I felt like I was about to be propelled into another situation where the expectations would be lowered for me. I feared that if I let that happen again, it would never end.

"I can take the test, Dr. Kelley!" I assured him.

With those words, he relented and gave me my test booklet and Scantron.

I started the test and immediately began to panic. None of the questions made sense. Besides Sir Gawain, I recognized none of the names or places mentioned in the questions. It was as if I had never read the book. I forced myself through that test, guessing the entire way. Thankfully, it was multiple choice. I just picked a letter and colored in the corresponding bubble on my Scantron. I handed in my test and left the classroom, wandering through the hall. I wanted to clear my head, but I also couldn't remember how to get back to the front of the school to meet Ryan so we could go home.

I ran into the Dean, David Cohen. He was startled by my bewildered look. He asked how I was feeling. I gave him the same answer I gave everyone else. I downplayed it.

"Fine, just a little sleepy," I said while my inner voice was screaming, *"I feel like crap! I'm pretty sure I just failed a test. I still can't feel the left side of my body and I really want to cry!"*

He couldn't even hear my inner voice and still suggested that I consider taking the rest of the semester off. He wanted me to leave school in the spring of my junior year and retake the classes when they were offered in the spring of 2004. I was supposed to graduate in the spring of 2004.

The difference between graduating in the spring of 2004 or the winter of 2004 likely seemed negligible to someone on the outside looking in. To me, though, it felt like the difference between struggling and quitting. My entire life had taught me to expect struggles. *Why would I have worked so hard at everything if quitting was an option, though?*

That's the exact reason why I make things sound less of a big deal. People always seemed to want to save me from the struggle. You cannot save me from the very foundation of my life. I realized that *I don't know who I am without the struggle.* My identity was tied to the concept of overcoming. If I did anything to make that year easier to get through, it would be to invalidate my entire college experience.

I remember the day Dr. Kelley was giving back the graded tests. He walked around the room and handed out the completed Scantrons. I held my breath, knowing I didn't do well but praying I didn't fail. The knot in my stomach got bigger with each student who looked at their score. I heard the sighs of relief and the whispers of "yes" all around me. I was praying that I would let out a similar sigh. Dr. Kelley walked up to me and held my Scantron out towards me. I could see the number written in red ink and circled. Within seconds, the tears came. *A 45?!*

"A freakin 45?" I muttered.

I didn't intend it to be audible, but it was. I took my test and wiped my eyes with the back of my hand. I wasn't about to cry in the middle of this class over a damn test! But it was the lowest grade I had ever gotten. I knew, logically, I should have offered myself some grace.

You had a stroke! You underwent 11 hours of neurosurgery! You spent five days in a coma, all AFTER reading that book. However, I wasn't in a headspace where I could be that kind to myself. All I could focus on was the failing grade. After class, Dr. Kelley pulled me aside.

"I won't count it. You can re-read it and re-take the test in a few weeks," he said. My professor was offering the compassion I couldn't even give myself.

"No! Count it! I'll make it up!" I told him.

My grades in that class had all been 100s or in the high 90s. I knew if I could pull off an A on the final, this 45 wouldn't damage my GPA too much. *Would I be able to do well on the final, though?*

I got home and I was still reeling from that 45. Mom asked me what was wrong. I held up the Scantron that I had crumpled up into a ball.

"This! This is wrong! I failed. I got a 45, mom!" I shouted and burst into tears.

Anything she said to try and console me fell flat. I was in the midst of a pity party that I had managed to go 23 years without failing. The culmination of decades of injuries, illnesses, and setbacks, when all I wanted to do was be normal, was finally coming to a head. I just sobbed. Mom just let me cry. I needed her to stop trying to make me feel better. Everything she said was logical, but all logic was lost on me. I just wanted to cry. She did just that. She let me cry.

She broke her silence and said, "Taniya, it was one test!"

How did she know it would stop at this test? Did she forget I still couldn't feel the left side of my body and was struggling to re-learn to tie my shoes?

I was a tornado of emotions and she just happened to be in my path when I replied.

"You don't know that it's only one test! We only know that it was this test! I still have a year's worth of tests I have to take before I graduate! What if I fail all those, too? What if I can't graduate?" I could no longer compose myself so mom offered me a tissue. There wasn't much she could do because I needed this catharsis. "If this is how the rest of my life is going to be, I wish you had let me die!"

She looked at me as if I had plunged a dagger through her heart. I immediately saw the pain in her eyes and felt awful. She bought me into this world. She had sacrificed so much for me to be standing before her right now. She had lost almost everything making sure I could have a life, and here I was, wishing she had let me die. She shouted back at me. Mom could outshout almost anyone.

"It's for now, not forever!" With that one sentence, she shut down my entire miserable pity party.

She was right. I was acting as if I was never going to recover, as if I could never get back to my baseline. *Had I truly forgotten all the times I had to recover before?* I had spent almost twenty years in a state of recovery. This wasn't uncharted territory for me. Why did it feel so different? Because I was trying to recover my mental faculties. I was accustomed to facing physical challenges. I was used to waiting for bones to heal. I could tolerate physical pain. But I was terrified that I wouldn't be able to overcome emotional pain and mental deficits. I defined myself by how intelligent I was. What would I have left if I was robbed of my intelligence and being physically disabled?

Every post-operative follow-up visit yielded no answers. *Why did I have s stroke at 23?* Nobody could make sense of that. When I asked when I could expect to get back to feeling like myself, I was told that "it will take time." How much time? Nobody knew. I wasn't asking for much. I just wanted to feel the left side of my body again. I wanted to understand and remember things I read. I wanted to not feel like I was going to fall over every time I stood up. I didn't want it to take me 15 minutes to put on my shoes anymore.

I once wanted to be "perfect." Now, I would have just settled for average.

It was a slow process. I stayed in school. I had to study twice as hard as I did before. I went to physical therapy three days a week for six months just to regain strength and feeling on the left side of my body. My peripheral vision in the left side never returned. Still, to this day, I have a problem with spatial relations. I can never tell how close or far I am in relation to something. I used to constantly walk into walls because I thought they were further away than they were. I would turn a corner and smack right into the corner of the wall. Those were just minor inconveniences in comparison to almost losing my whole life.

In May of 2004, a little over a year after my stroke, I graduated from college. I graduated Summa Cum Laude with a Bachelor's in Fine Arts. I was aiming for valedictorian. I fell just a tad short, but I graduated as a straight-A student! No special education classes. No accommodations. No extra time on tests and exemptions from anything physical. I did that! A few days before graduation, the Dean, who suggested I take the semester off after my stroke, called me to his office. I expected he wanted to talk about the logistics of graduation. The ceremony would take place in the theater, which was still inaccessible. I thought he was going to talk about how to get me up to the stage to get my diploma. I was prepared to tell him that I'd been navigating the school for the past four years and that I'd figure out graduation day. He surprised me. He didn't call there to talk about my graduation day strategy. He told me he was proud of me.

"I didn't think you'd be able to pull this off," he said.

I already knew that. A year ago, nobody thought I would be days from graduation. That was probably one of the only reasons I did. Doubt I can do something, and I'll do it three times and send you directions. He said I was an inspiration.

I'd been called an inspiration before, but this time, it hit differently. I actually *did* something to be inspired by. I worked my ass off to come back from the biggest setback of my life. When everyone said to give up, I let that fuel my determination and pushed forward. At that time, that was the hardest year of my life. It's not every day you get to stare down death, so it was also the most fulling year of my life. I was damn proud of myself.

I walked across the stage at graduation as the physical manifestation of everything people told me I couldn't be or do. I was an adult, a college graduate, an honor student, and I was walking.

After my stroke, I had this nagging fear that I was going to die young. I was most afraid that I would come close to dying, be on life support, and mom just leave me like that. I was almost ashamed that a year earlier, I looked her in the face and told her she should have let me die. We sat at the kitchen table late one night and I made her promise that if I ever ended up on life support, she wouldn't leave me to be a vegetable, but she wouldn't give up on me too early.

"Mom, if anything happens to me and I'm not breathing on life support, wait for a sign, unless doctors tell you I'm brain dead. I'll let you know if I'm not coming back. Look for a sign from me," I told her.

I explained that living on life support is no life I would want. Naturally, she knew if I was brain dead, I'd be trapped in my worst nightmare. She nodded and agreed. I thought that was the end of the conversation until she looked at me and said, "Promise you'll do the same for me." At the time, I couldn't think of my mom in terms of *end-of-life* decisions. At the time, she was only 48. But, later, it would be a conversation I am so glad that we had.

Girl, Don't Beg For Love

Ryan was one of my best friends in college. He supported me through my stroke recovery. He was kind and understanding. He brought me food and walked me to and from classes when I couldn't remember how to get there. He was exactly what I needed at that time. With my freshly bald head and skinny frame — I had dropped so much weight — I needed someone to call me beautiful. I needed someone to make me feel special and cared for when my life felt like it was falling apart.

I want to say that he led me on, but that's not a fair statement. I led myself on by ignoring anything that didn't fit the narrative that I was trying to create. Had I given myself all the attention and affection I showered him with, I would have known that I deserved more than a half-hearted relationship. I would have demanded that he go all in or go away. I feel bad for that 24-year-old girl. She was willing to settle for half of love instead of learning to love herself fully. She was willing to beg and grovel to be loved. I remember the exact moment Ryan was finally honest with himself and with me.

"I love you, but I can't be with you. I'm too superficial for you," Ryan eventually said.

Instead of turning on my heels and walking away, I started running off the list of all the things I was.

"But I'm smart, funny, kind, caring. I love you …" I said, until I ran out of breath.

I was trying to convince a man that I was good enough. I felt compelled to prove I was more than the Little Person with a bald head and deformed limbs.

I'm too superficial for you. That played on every insecurity I had as a disabled woman. *What defines beauty? Does beauty require two equally working legs? Is beauty tall with long, flowing hair?* I knew Ryan's dream girl was a dancer. He loved a dancer's body, and we were surrounded by them. He wanted something that I could never be. That was a reality that I had to face. I tried so hard to be everything he would want. I spent our entire relationship changing who I was in order to be what I perceived he wanted.

Shortly after my stroke, Ryan moved. He transferred to a school in Pennsylvania. We kept in touch, and I visited him once or twice a month, but those visits became less frequent. I needed the space. I wanted to learn how to unlove someone who didn't want me. I deserved to be desired and wanted. I don't know if I wanted him nearly as much as I just wanted him to want me. As if his having some primal sexual attraction to me would magically create some sense of self-worth for me. If the object of my desire also desired me, I thought it would leave me feeling sexy, beautiful, and confident.

I was great at faking confidence, but I had none. Everyone who knew me at that time thought I was the most confident and self-assured woman. In reality, I was just a brilliant actress. The greatest performance of my life was acting like I didn't have insecurities. I was great at pretending to be all the things I wished I was. But I knew I couldn't act my way into a normal body. So I feigned my way into a confident mindset.

If I'm honest with myself, I wouldn't have dated the 24-year-old version of myself. She needed constant validation. She was searching for someone to complete her. Nothing about that is attractive. The thing my 24-year-old self needed most was to learn how to be whole on her own before seeking love from someone else. Self-love didn't come naturally to me, and I grew up way before daily affirmations were commonplace. It felt awkward to think of myself as beautiful. I was ashamed when I thought about myself positively. I perceived being complimentary to myself as someone who is conceited. I was raised to believe you let people compliment you, and you graciously accept them, but you never compliment yourself.

When the few states between Ryan and I began to feel like galaxies away, it was clear we had to cut ties entirely. I'd call. He wouldn't answer or return my call. My feelings would be hurt, but I'd call again 24 hours later and the same thing would happen. I noticed the pattern and I knew it was unhealthy. I had to let go, and to do that, I had to remind myself of how terrible I felt when he said, "I can't be with you. I'm too superficial for you." Like pouring salt on a gaping wound. I needed it to hurt so I could release what I thought was love. I didn't want to picture our children when I thought of him. Replacing the positive imagery with the painful reality hurt like hell, but it worked.

It would be easy to look back at that time with regret. Sure, I wasted a lot of time. I poured myself into the relationship I wanted with complete tunnel vision. I gave more than I knew I'd ever get in return.

I'm unbelievably filled with gratitude for Ryan and that relationship. He taught me one of the most important lessons I ever learned: I should never have to beg for love. If it's not a love given freely and equally, it's not a love worth having. It's painful to admit that I was begging. I wasn't just begging to be loved, though. I was also begging to feel worthy and deserving of love. That's something no relationship could ever give me. It was something I eventually found when I took the time and looked inward. Feeling worthy and deserving is not one of the *bells and whistles* you get with a relationship. It's found in solitude and quiet reflection on yourself. I will never again beg for love.

You Can Mend A Broken Heart

I'm not one to say, "What else can go wrong?" Because I've learned that the universe will always find something else, even when you least expect it. I was living a fairly unassuming post-college life — working full-time, looking for theater gigs, and paying back student loans. It was a relatively normal life for a 25-year-old. I enjoyed the normalcy. I naively thought the worst was behind me. I was walking almost full-time. I hadn't broken anything since high school. I had no major long-term impact from the stroke. By every measure, I was doing well. I had survived well past my "expiration date." I had overcome everything that God threw at me. Living through my stroke made me feel a bit invincible. At the very least I knew God didn't want me yet. I had things to accomplish. Otherwise, why would he have left me here?

It was a cold winter day, the week before Christmas. We were expecting a snowstorm. In New York snow is quite common. I had plans with my best friend from high school, Alex. Alex was my rock. After college, we worked together and still made plans to hang out on weekends. She'd been with me through everything. We were grown women and still as close as we were in high school. To this day, she's still my very best friend.

That day, I went over to her house to build gingerbread houses. I felt fine all day. Alex said I looked fine, and I didn't complain about not feeling well.

When I left her house, it started to snow. It was light snow at first, barely covering the streets, but it got heavier quickly. I started to panic. A feeling of terror swept over me. I couldn't think straight. I was terribly panicked. Extreme weather always caused me to panic. During thunderstorms, if there was lightning, I'd hide in the hallway away from all the windows. Before I knew it, I was lost. I was in the town I went to high school in. I knew all the landmarks like the back of my hand: the high school, the bagel store, the post office, the diner. I'd been to all those places dozens of times, but nothing looked familiar. I called my parents and Alex asking for directions.

"Tell me what you see," they all said, trying to pinpoint my location.

I was zero help because I started hallucinating.

"A purple house," I said.

Mom immediately turned to Google searching "Purple houses in Mount Sinai."

Next, I saw a police department. There are no police departments in Mount Sinai. Next, I thought I saw a police car behind me. Mom called all the precincts trying to find out if my 1995 Dodge Neon had been pulled over. When I said, "I see an elephant crossing the street," I hung up the phone to watch the elephant. To my mom, the line went dead and it was obvious that something was terribly wrong.

The last thing I remember about that day is seeing that elephant walking across the street only feet away from my car. I had no clue I was hallucinating. It felt so real. Mom had said she became concerned that Alex and I had used psychedelic drugs. From her experience with the police department, the only time she saw people hallucinating was when they were on drugs. Mom should have known better. I'd never touched a drug in my life. Alex and I were "good kids."

I woke up that night in the hospital. I was hooked up to every monitor they had, oxygen shooting up my nose and everyone was staring at me.

"What happened?" I asked.

This was starting to get really old. *Was passing out and waking up in the hospital my new version of breaking a bone?*

"You were in a car accident," Mom told me.

"Did I hit the elephant?" I asked.

Once I heard the words escape my lips, I realized how insane that question sounded and wished I could take it back. I was flooded with questions from everyone in the room.

"How much did you have to drink today?"

"Have you used any recreational drugs?"

"Do you take any prescription drugs?"

"No. No. And only if you count the Prilosec I take for chronic heartburn," I answered.

I was in a car accident. People get in car accidents every day, especially in a snowstorm. *Why was I being interrogated?*

The toxicology test came back and proved that my system was clean. I heard the story of what happened, about all the phone calls I had made and the things I said I was seeing. I remembered the purple house and the elephant, but was shocked by everything else. I didn't even remember spending the day with Alex. It started to snow, but had no clue when or where I got lost. A cop saw me drive my car off the road and into the woods. I was about two towns away from where I had started. I hit a tree and was found unconscious.

They did a series of CAT scans and said they saw nothing of concern. It was déjà vu. I'd heard that before. The doctor said I had a mild concussion, most likely from the impact of the accident. That was plausible but didn't explain the hallucinations. Doctors were grasping at straws. I heard everything from I possibly didn't get enough sleep the night before to some undiagnosed form of mental illness. I'm still not sure if they even looked at my history of brain trauma. They should have. I was in the same hospital that saved my life the night of my stroke.

The cardiologist walked in carrying the reports from my EKG and echocardiogram. They did those tests for good measure. On the off chance I had a heart attack, they'd be able to tell. The cardiologist had an intense look on his face. I could see he was having a "Eureka!" moment.

"Taniya, do you have mitral valve prolapse?" he asked.

Why was he asking me? He was holding the tests that would tell him definitively.

"Yes. I've had it my whole life," I told him. I really didn't feel like going through my extensive health history because of a car accident.

"That's it!" he declared.

This was starting to feel like a poorly written medical TV show. If I didn't know better, I would have thought he was auditioning for the latest season of *Grey's Anatomy*. Mom stared at him. I knew that look on her face. That was her *get-to-the-point* face. She was not one to listen to my doctors beat around the bush. I was less intrigued. The last thing I wanted was to be diagnosed with something else. I didn't want another disorder, disease, or medical anomaly to disrupt the normalcy I had to work so hard to achieve.

"Your mitral valve is leaking so much that not enough blood is getting to your brain. That's why you passed out," he said.

He further explained that when the brain is devoid of proper oxygenation, the person can have visions and see things that aren't there.

He suggested that I follow up with a heart surgeon to discuss options for having my mitral valve repaired. I knew my body. After all, I had recognized a bleeding brain that nobody saw. If my brain was being deprived of oxygen, I would be the first to know. I thought that the doctor was nuts.

I was born with mitral valve prolapse. It ran in our family. Mom and grandma had it. It wasn't something I ever had to think about. It was always checked during my yearly physicals. I saw a cardiologist periodically. I was never told it could or would be a problem. I certainly never heard that it would cause me to pass out. I was convinced this doctor didn't know what he was talking about but I obliged and said I would follow up with a cardiologist. I really didn't want to, but mom was all in. She wasn't going to let me off the hook.

When I saw my cardiologist, I fully expected that he would agree with me. I had no symptoms he would expect to see in someone with heart problems. I didn't have shortness of breath, palpitations, or chest pain. Although I knew MVP was fairly unassuming, it just felt pretty far-fetched that after 20-plus years of causing me no problems, it was suddenly causing me to pass out. Unfortunately, he didn't agree with me. He ordered a new echocardiogram. I've had those before. I never understood how they are useful. They just produce a grainy image of what is supposed to be the heart. They are not nearly as clear as the X-rays I used to see. But cardiologists love them. He came back carrying several pieces of paper. He had a very focused look on his face.

"The valve is pretty weak," he said. "You see this piece right here?" he asked as he showed me a very blurry gray and white printout. It reminded me of the printout of sonograms that pregnant women are given. I nodded, although I didn't see the piece he was talking about.

"This is supposed to be here," he continued, as he pointed to another area.

I couldn't make heads or tails of what he was showing me. Maybe I shouldn't have, but I just stopped listening to him. I'm normally a very active participant in my health care, but I was tired. I wasn't tired only on that day, but I was tired in general. How many tests, X-rays, CAT scans, or MRIs did I have to listen the results of? I wanted no part of it anymore. It started to feel as if the more they tested me, the more they ultimately found was wrong.

"Yes," I told him with growing frustration.

"That's your mitral valve and it's really not closing anymore. You are getting a significant backflow into your heart."

They didn't just *find* something wrong. They went *looking* for something to diagnose. It's like the old adage, "Seek and ye shall find." He referred me to a cardiothoracic surgeon in Manhattan.

It had been ages since I last traveled to New York City for medical care. Outside of my stroke, I hadn't needed any specialized medical care. I met Dr. Loulmet at his office in Manhattan. He was affiliated with Lenox Hill Hospital, one of the premier hospitals in New York. His list of credentials was lengthy and diverse. One of his most impressive was that he could perform surgery with the assistance of a robotic "arm." The science nerd in me thought that was the coolest thing ever. This man could use a robot to do heart surgery. Logistically, it made sense. Being a Little Person, I have a small chest cavity. Because of my OI, I have an oddly shaped sternum and rib cage, giving it a unique barrel shape. So, thinking about a tiny robot arm working on my heart was much more appealing than imagining two large man-sized hands in there. Dr. Loulmet agreed that my mitral valve should be repaired at some point. He thought this was the perfect time to do it, citing my age.

"You're 24. You'll recover quicker than you will at 50 or 60," he said.

That was a matter of fact I couldn't dispute. I wanted to find any excuse to put off the surgery, but there wasn't one. If I needed surgery, might as well just get it over with. I was finished with school. I was working a full-time job that offered me a full salary while I took a medical leave of absence. Dr. Loulmet made a lot of promises that felt too good to be true: three days in the hospital, three weeks before I could return to work, a "tiny" scar from a single incision he would need to make, and a mitral valve repair instead of a full replacement. He was confident my valve could be salvaged.

I was scared as hell but I gave in. I committed to the surgery. It terrified me that in order to perform the surgery, they would need to stop my heart. *What if they couldn't get it to start again? What if I never woke up? What if I died because of an elective surgery?* My faith was always super strong. I had an unwavering belief in God. Sometimes I questioned his decisions and wished he hadn't put so much on me. But I never questioned his existence. I knew if my time was up on this planet, he could have taken me in 2003 when I had my stroke.

I went back to that feeling of invincibility I had after my stroke when I learned I cheated death that night. I reminded myself God was in control. He didn't place such a brilliant surgeon in my path without some divine plan for this ending well. I had to believe that. I scheduled my surgery for April 5, 2005, exactly two years and two days after another brilliant surgeon operated on me and successfully saved my life. I was confident April was a good month.

The day before the surgery, I felt nervous. I had this nagging feeling that I was going to die. That was something I wasn't used to feeling. I'm used to being optimistic. I'm used to being secure that every broken bone and surgery has a purpose and ends well. I remembered the uncertainty of childhood — the days when I just kept breaking bones and no one knew why. No one knew how or when my story ends. Right now, I feel the same uncertainty that I felt at 5 years old. But right now, there were no coloring books or cartoons to distract me. I retreated to my room to talk to God. I need to do more than just pray. I sat in the middle of the floor and started talking. We didn't go to church often. We joked that mom was the worst Roman Catholic ever. She rarely took us to church. Mom always told me, "God is where you are." I'd only been to confession once, right before my first Holy Communion. I think you were supposed to apologize for everything you did wrong. I couldn't remember if I was allowed to ask for anything besides forgiveness. I just opened my mouth and started talking. It was one stream of consciousness.

"God, I don't know how much more you can ask me to go through. Haven't I met every challenge you put before me? Why do you keep pushing me to the point of death?" I asked. "What is it you want from me?"

The challenges always felt the same, as if I was being asked to do something more than just persevere.

"What lesson haven't I learned?" I continued.

Obviously, he didn't answer, so I resorted to barter with God. The offers I made were the same types of deals I'd make with mom when I was a kid. If I asked her to stay up later at night, I'd offer to do an extra chore.

"God, if you just let me survive tomorrow, I'll do whatever I have to in order to make this world a better place. If you let me live past 25, I'll use the time wisely. I'll serve you, I promise."

I looked around the room for some sign or signal. Out of the corner of my left eye, I saw a glowing yellowish orb. I have a huge blind spot in the periphery of my left eye. I normally don't see anything there. That's why ever since my stroke, I walk into walls on the left side. To suddenly have vision and see this ball of light unnerved me. I questioned if I was seeing God. Spirits and God appear as light, right? I vaguely remembered a prayer that said, "God is light."

I left my dark room and went into my parents' room. I wanted to be around people. If I wasn't hallucinating, mom and dad would see this orb too. I heard Ashley in there as well. Ashley can be dramatic, so I knew if she didn't see this orb, it definitely wasn't there. I didn't know if this yellow orb was a good or bad sign, but I feel it was a sign. I just started talking. I was saying my goodbyes. I was convinced I was going to die in the morning. I wondered if this is the "white light" people say they see as they die. What if it starts out yellow and turns white as you die? I started telling them that I hoped I was a good daughter and how much I loved them. I knew Ashley and I didn't always get along, but I hoped in death she would remember me as a good sister. I was convinced this was my last night on this planet and I wanted to leave them with something. I wanted them to know all the things I may not have ever said to them. Then, another orb joined the yellow one. This one was blue and flashing. It had a rhythm to its flashing. It was almost like the lights I would see when I went to clubs during my college years. I got confused and couldn't make the words I wanted to say come out of my mouth. Mom described it by saying I sounded like an electronic doll malfunctioning. I was trying to say the word die but I got stuck on the letter "D" and said "Da Da Da" until I passed out.

My parents immediately took me to the emergency room. I regained consciousness relatively quickly. The minute I woke up I thought I was in the recovery room and my heart surgery was complete. I was relieved that I had lived through it. I started thanking God and mom broke the news to me that surgery hadn't happened yet. I remembered talking to God. I remembered seeing the glowing orbs, but nothing beyond that. The doctors were unsure what had happened. Everything looked fine. They called it a panic attack due to the extreme stress of worrying about the surgery. Mom called Dr. Loulmet's office and everybody agreed that we should delay the surgery for at least a week. *Great! Just want I wanted — an additional week to worry about this surgery.*

My heart surgery took place two weeks later. Like something out of a Sci-Fi movie, Dr. Loulmet cooled my heart down to the point it stopped beating. I was placed on a heart lung machine that circulated my blood and breathed for me while Dr. Loulmet used wire and a plastic ring to repair my mitral valve so it would close completely. Once it was repaired, he warmed my heart up until it started beating again and placed it back in my chest. Once surgery was complete, I was extubated. My heart was beating and I was breathing on my own. I am still in awe of the science behind that surgery.

That recovery was by far my easiest. Almost *too* easy. I spent three days in the hospital and returned home. I couldn't believe I was so fearful of something that felt so simple after the fact. The worst part was the healing my broken sternum had to go through. To get to my heart, Dr. Loulmet had to use a bone saw and rib spreader to open my chest. Every breath, every cough, and every sneeze made my chest feel like it was bursting open. Outside of that, I almost forgot I had it done.

Perhaps, the fact that my stroke recovery was so grueling made heart surgery feel so simple. Regardless, I was relieved that it was so "easy."

Even though my heart was fixed, I continued to have episodes that would lead to me passing out. Sometimes I'd see things just as peculiar as the elephant I saw walk across the street before my car accident. Other times, I just couldn't speak. All these episodes always ended the same: I'd lose consciousness, sleep for hours, and often struggled to remember want had happened. I saw multiple doctors and no one could diagnose the problem. I'd randomly feel dizzy. I saw family members who had passed away. I saw flashing lights, most notably in my peripheral vision. I'd hear continuous ringing in my ears. The left side of my face would feel numb. I had severe anxiety and full-blown panic attacks. Doctors were really quick to revisit their favorite diagnosis for me: they thought I was mentally ill. No one discussed mental illness with me but every chance they got, they recommended I see a psychiatrist.

I was over it. I was tired of seeing doctors for symptoms that no one understood. I was sick of talking about my childhood to psychiatrists. It felt like they were all waiting for me to say something that would allow them to diagnose what was happening as some form of schizophrenia that they could medicate away. One psychiatrist had the audacity to ask me if I was sexually abused as a child. I remember this line of questioning. Twenty years ago, when no one knew why my bones were breaking, they tried to blame my parents. I knew my body well enough to know these episodes were very real. I saw, heard, and felt things as very real as I saw, heard, or felt members of my family. I was fed up with screaming, "Stop dismissing me! Somebody please help me!"

I heard it all. I heard ocular migraines, stress headaches, high blood pressure, low blood sugar, anxiety, and panic disorders.

Finally, right before my psychiatrist announced he would increase my Xanax, he said, "What if the problem is neurological and not emotional?"

Was he asking me or telling me? Or was he just thinking out loud? I wasn't sure, but until that point, nobody looked for an underlying neurological cause.

He referred me to a neurologist. I hated all of them. I went through about eight neurologists. I found them smug and way too scientific when they spoke. At times, I felt like they were speaking at me and not to me. Being physically disabled, I'm used to people talking at me. It still makes me just as angry as it did when I was five. So every time a neurologist would pose that as a possibility, I'd leave his office and never come back. I'd make an appointment with a different neurologist for a second opinion. That second opinion became a third and fourth opinion. They all landed on the same theory: I had epilepsy as a result of the stroke.

I thought that it was another shot-in-the-dark diagnosis to explain something nobody had been able to diagnose. I couldn't have epilepsy. I played video games, went to night clubs with strobe lights and fog machines, and had none of these episodes. No one had ever seen me have convulsions. No one could confirm any shaking, foaming at the mouth, or "swallowing" my tongue while I was caught in these episodes. Everyone who witnessed these described the same thing: an electronic doll or toy robot with a dying battery. My speech would slow down, and then I'd get "stuck" on one syllable or sound until I passed out. Afterwards, I'd sleep for hours, but when I woke up, I'd still feel exhausted.

Unfortunately, I had an antiquated idea of what epilepsy looked like. The result was that I rebuked every doctor who even uttered the word to me. Also, I didn't want another diagnosis. I didn't think I could handle something else being wrong with me. It wasn't self-pity as much as it was frustration. I had wracked up 100 broken bones, had a stroke, neurosurgery, and heart surgery, and I was only 25! I didn't want to add another specialist to the growing list of doctors I saw.

I finally submitted to a battery of tests, most of which were horrific. I underwent several EEGs. Multiple electrodes were glued to my scalp, and my head was wrapped in a layer of gauze to measure my brain waves and look for any electrical abnormalities. I was kept awake for 24 hours, had a strobe light flashed in my face, and was endlessly questioned all while I was in the hospital. I did a 24-hour EEG session where I'd be confined to one room and videotaped the entire time. The only time I was off camera was if I went into the bathroom. Otherwise, they were always watching me, looking for any physical manifestation of seizure activity happening in my brain. I felt like a fish in a fishbowl just being stared at, waiting for it to do something.

When the results came in, they were not inconclusive at all. I had hoped they would be. It was definitive. I was epileptic. I had officially been diagnosed with complex partial seizures that originated in my right temporal lobe. It is not a coincidence that the right temporal lobe was the site of the original bleeding. The rouge electrical impulses that would start in the right temporal lobe would quickly run into the occipital parietal lobes, causing the visual hallucinations and the loss of consciousness. I sometimes wonder if the glowing orbs that I saw during my seizures are my mind's eye seeing the electricity going haywire in my brain.

They threw numerous anti-epileptic drugs at me: Tegretol, Depakote, Dilantin, Phenobarbital, Lamictal, Vimpat, and Keppra. Most were not well tolerated by my system. Tegretol and Depakote made me feel like a zombie. Phenobarbital made me insanely nauseous. Dilantin and Vimpat gave me really weird dreams. Most days, I just didn't feel like myself. In spite of all the medication, my seizures persisted.

The most frustrating part was when I would spend 10 minutes in the morning and again before bed trying to choke down multiple pills, only to continue to have several seizures a week. My doctors would charge my medication, increase or decrease the dose, or invent a new cocktail for me to try, but nothing stopped my seizures. Out of complacency, and because I was so worn out, I just accepted this was how the rest of my life was going to be. I wasn't giving up, but I had very little fight left, so I had to surrender. I gave it to God and prayed that he would bring me through this.

If he brings you to it, he will bring you through it...

God was about to change our household forever. In 2007, Ashley announced that she was pregnant. To think my baby sister was going to have a baby blew my mind more than any seizure ever could. "A girl," she told us. Not only was I going to be an aunt, but I was going to be an aunt to a little girl. Mom had her concerns, but she was excited too. She and dad were about to be grandparents. We all still lived in one house together. It was only a three-bedroom house, so it wasn't ideal, but we were the family who lived in a motel for four years, after all. Certainly, we could handle the addition of a baby when we were living in a whole house. The last time there was a child in our family was when Tevon was with us. It was exciting to think that this little baby would one day be 3 years old like he was. I remembered how much I loved having him around. I'd get to teach my niece things and watch her grow up. That was going to be a lot of fun.

Ashley and I share genetics. We are biological sisters. Ashley did not have OI. Neither did anyone in our family that we knew of. There was no way to tell how or why I was born with OI. Silently, I worried about Ashley's baby.

What if there's a gene for OI that gets passed on to the baby?

Gianna was born July 4, 2008. She was just as fiercely independent as her birthday suggests.

"I will give you one year to get things together," Mom told Ashley. Ashley was a young, single mom living with her parents. Mom's one-year timeline seemed perfectly reasonable. At the time, Ashley didn't realize that wasn't a timeline. It was a deadline.

It's For Now, Not Forever

I inherited my mitral valve prolapse from my mom. She got it from her mother. For as long as I can remember, we were three generations of women, all cursed with the same affliction. Mine was now repaired. Grandma's never seemed to cause her any problems. I'm not sure she even had to see a cardiologist. I now only had to follow up with one once a year. My heart was often called a "perfect repair." My cardiologist talked about how *beautiful* my repair looked on imaging and how well my heart functioned. I remember at one of my visits, he told me that most people can only hope for a repair this good. He didn't intend it to be, but there was a level of foreshadowing in that statement that I would never see coming.

Out of the three of us, mom's heart gave her the most trouble. It's not surprising. She was a moderate cigarette smoker. She was continuously under stress trying to juggle all her balls in the air without ever fumbling. As she got older, she gained weight and had high blood pressure, a fairly common problem in America. She was on medication to control her blood pressure and never missed it. She was not the healthiest person in the world, but she wasn't sick either. I was the sick one in the family! By all accounts, she was just a suburban mother: two kids, a husband, a full-time job, and eating on the go with little time for self-care. She always put others before herself. So when the choice was to make a home-cooked meal for her family or work out for an hour, she'd always pick doing things for her family. That's just who she was.

She was taken to the emergency room several times for bouts of angina and tachycardia. She was always treated and released with discharge notes that told her to quit smoking and lose weight. Ironically enough, after my heart surgery, her cardiac incidents seemed to increase. She still never seemed sick, just subtly annoyed. She rarely complained, but would occasionally mention she was having chest pains or shortness of breath. I love my mom for how much she cared for Ashley and me. We never missed doctor's appointments. She'd go to the 24-hour pharmacy at midnight looking for Tylenol at the first signs we had a fever. She gave endlessly, often putting herself last. I sometimes wonder if she intentionally put herself last or just got so caught up in caring for others that she forgot about herself.

After leaving work early to go to the emergency room because she was having chest pains again, mom followed up with her cardiologist. She was given the vague diagnosis of early stage heart disease. She already knew that. She had complied with doctor's orders. She lost weight, took her high blood pressure medication regularly, and ate well. Much to dad's dismay, she cut out all red meat. The woman was eating grilled chicken and kale salads. It wasn't enough. Her blood pressure was stable but her heart was strained. The doctor believed that her mitral valve was leaking and it put undue stress on her already diseased heart. His recommendation was to have her mitral valve repaired. When she told me, I wasn't surprised. I was given the same advice four years earlier and had it done. It seemed commonplace.

Mom met with several surgeons. She was hesitant to move forward with the surgery. She met with my surgeon, Dr. Loulmet, but he couldn't do her surgery. He had a few conferences lined up, and after those, he was booked solid. He referred her to another Manhattan cardiothoracic surgeon. When she met with that doctor, she came home and said, "I think I found my surgeon." I was happy for her. I knew firsthand how important it is to trust your surgeon. You walk into every surgery knowing you don't have to come out of the operating room alive. It's the surgeon's job to make sure that you do. I've been blessed with surgeons that I have always trusted and adored.

She scheduled her surgery for early April, and I told her, "April is a good month for surgery!" It was in April that I had my life-saving neurosurgery. I also had my mitral valve repair done in April, exactly four years earlier. I had an affinity for that month. Call it superstition, but I thought no surgery could go wrong if it was done in April. Mom was hesitant but committed to just getting it over with.

In the weeks leading up to her surgery, she asked me so many questions about my recovery. She didn't have to ask because she saw it firsthand. I lived with her during all my surgeries. Maybe she thought I downplayed the depth of pain and the toll that recovery took on me. I told her it was no big deal. Looking back, I probably should have said that for me, it was no big deal. No one should use me as a barometer for how easy or hard anything is. My pain tolerance is above average. There's no way to break bones every few weeks for years without unknowingly building an extreme tolerance for pain. Physically, mentally, and emotionally I have been forced to endure more than most people. So it's easy for me to scoff at a surgery or procedure and call it "no big deal." I really wish I hadn't.

Mom had an intense fear that she might die during surgery. In an effort to allay her fears, I told her this surgery was common. I pointed out how quickly I recovered. She knew the surgery itself only took a few hours because she had to wait for me during mine. I made silly jokes.

"We'll have matching scars. You know you want to join the zipper club!" I told her, referring to the scar that runs down the center of my chest which resembles a zipper.

Phrases like, "It'll be fine, mom," and "You got this," were offered up as words of encouragement.

She'd reply with a half-hearted, "You're right."

I wanted her to be confident. I needed her to go into surgery with a positive mindset. Her faith was strong. I expected her to just trust God. For whatever reason, she didn't, and I just kept trying to build her confidence in science, medicine, and doctors. I know that's what she would have done for me. Any time I didn't want a medical test, cast, or procedure, she'd build up my confidence in why it was important and tell me how easy it would be.

A few nights before her surgery, she and I stayed up late chatting in the kitchen.

"How do they know you're dead before they bury you?" she asked me.

I knew that was a rhetorical question that didn't require a response, but I responded anyway.

"Mom, they check for a heartbeat, pulse, and unassisted breathing."

She stared at me unmoved.

"Also, there are several days between when a person dies and the burial," I continued. "If the person was still alive, somewhere between the morgue and funeral home, they'd wake up or someone would notice them breathing," I said before realizing she wasn't really asking the question.

She was covertly expressing *I'm afraid I'm going to die.* We stared at each other for what felt like an eternity, but it couldn't have been more than 45 seconds. The clock behind her never moved from 10:33 to 10:34. I will never forget those 45 seconds that I spent trying to subliminally convince her she was not going to die. I still wonder if that stare swayed her decision.

My infallible, unshakable warrior goddess of a mother was afraid she was going to die? I couldn't make sense of that. She seemingly had no fears. She was the strongest person I knew. I couldn't reconcile that she was afraid.

I decided to go to work the morning of her surgery. Dad was going to take her. I had just accepted a job closer to my house. I wasn't doing life-altering work, but I didn't want to miss any time. She would have never done that to me. Mom was always the last face I saw before being rolled into an operating room. I denied her that same level of support because I had to go to a job that would end up firing me three months later. I hugged her and gave her a kiss.

"You got this!" I said. I looked at my dad and nodded. A silent signal to keep being supportive.

Support was never my dad's strong suit.

"Call me when she gets out," I added. He nodded back, and they left.

I waited for that call to come. I checked my phone every few minutes. Those minutes felt like hours. *Where were they?* I hadn't heard from dad since early morning when he told me they had just taken her into surgery. It was now lunch and he still hadn't called. My mind was racing. I called my dad multiple times and he didn't answer. That was not unlike my father. Still to this day, he doesn't answer his cell phone. I was getting anxious. *What if something had happened to her?* No matter how easy a surgery feels after the fact, they all carry the risk of complications. I called my sister, who was at the house with Gianna, who was 9 months old at the time.

"Have you heard from dad yet?" I asked her.

"No, he hasn't called yet. It's fine, Taniya. It's just taking longer than yours," she told me.

I knew she was right. When I had mine done, I was half my mother's age. Maybe I was just a quick fix. Shortly before I was set to leave work, the call came. I saw it was my father and answered with nervous anticipation.

"Is she out?" I quickly asked. I knew if I left it up to him, he would tell me some long drawn-out story before getting to what I really needed to know.

"She's out. She's in the cardiac ICU. She'll be there for the night. Tomorrow, they'll move her to the step-down unit. If she does well there, she can come home in three or four days."

Who the hell was this man on the other end of my phone? My father never gets all the information. How did he know so much? He barely listens to anyone who speaks to him. Yet somehow, he managed to hear and remember all of this?! He told me he was going to catch the next train out of Penn Station and would tell me more when he got home. With that, I left work and headed home.

I had just gotten in the house and out of my work clothes before the phone rang. *Who was calling the house?* Me, Ashley, and dad all had cellphones. Rarely did we get calls on the home phone. I answered it.

"Can I speak to Mr. Lamont Faulk?" I thought it was a solicitor and was annoyed by the call.

"Mr. Faulk is not home. His wife just had surgery today!" I said as snippy as possible.

"I know. I'm calling from Mount Sinai Hospital."

My mind started racing. Mount Sinai Hospital is the hospital where mom had surgery. Why were they calling? Why were they looking for dad?

"What happened?" I asked.

"Ma'am, I need to speak to Mr. Faulk. I tried him on his cellphone, but he didn't answer."

I wasn't surprised, dad never answers his cell phone.

"What happened?" I asked again, my stomach in a knot.

"Ma'am, I need to speak with her husband. He's her next of kin."

I tried to take a deep breath. Deep breathing was how I battled anxiety every day, but right now, it was as if I had forgotten how to breathe. *Why did she need to speak to her next of kin? Was this woman calling to tell dad that my mom had just died? She was fine a few hours ago.*

"Lamont Faulk is on the train headed home. He just left my mom. She was in the cardiac ICU recovering. What happened?"

"Ma'am, I don't know if we have a signed HIPAA release. Please have your father call the hospital and ask to be transferred to the nurse's station of the Cardiac ICU."

I grew more nervous with each breath. I knew this call meant something bad.

"Lady, my dad is on the train as we speak. It will take him at least 90 minutes to make it back to Long Island. I won't see him for two hours. Please just tell me!" I begged, my voice quivering. I know she heard the desperation in my voice. Suddenly she wasn't worried about a HIPAA anymore.

"Right after your dad left, your mom went into cardiac arrest. Her heart did stop, but they were able to restart it," she said. I don't know why, but her use of the word "they" bothered me. "They" could be a doctor, nurse, the janitor.

"Who's they?" I shouted into the phone.

"The surgeon. Your mom just had surgery. The surgeon went back in. He was able to perform an open-heart massage and got her heart restarted." I wanted to feel relieved, but I didn't. I wouldn't feel relief until I saw her. "She's doing well now. She's asleep," the nurse said.

My mind flooded with thoughts that I struggled to keep track of. *Was she afraid? Does she have an awareness of what she went through? Is she in pain? Does she know where she is? Is she wondering where her family is? What happens next? She's sleeping now, but what about tomorrow? Is she breathing on her own? Was this a setback or could her recovery still go as planned?*

I wanted to be with her. I needed her to know she wasn't alone. She deserved the same support she always gave me when I was in the hospital. It would be impossible to get to her that night. By the time dad made it home and we got back to the train station, and took the train into Penn Station, it would be after visiting hours. I knew that. It was clear the earliest I would get to see mom would be the next morning.

I wished I wasn't the one to take that call because now it was my responsibility to relay this information to Ashley and dad. I didn't even want to say the words *mom's heart stopped.* So I certainly didn't want to recall all the details out loud. Ashley was home with me when I took the call. She was only a room away. I wasn't certain what, if anything, she overheard. I knew that I had to be delicate when I told her. She was still my little sister. That instinct to protect her had always been a huge part of our dynamic. She also had an infant daughter to care for. I didn't want to inflict undue worry on her, so I downplayed it.

"Mom's okay!" That was my buffer. "But she had a heart attack. The doctors were able to restart her heart though. She's fine," I concluded. I threw the last line in more for myself than for Ashley. I wanted to hear that our mother was fine.

We took turns trying to call dad. He kept letting the calls go to voicemail. This wasn't the kind of thing you just left on someone's voicemail. He didn't need to know this minute anyway. *What was he going to do? Tell the train to turn around and take him back to the city?* He still had a 20-minute drive home once he got back to Long Island. I needed him to make it home safely before I told him. The truest fact about my father is that he does not perform well under stress, especially stress related to medical concerns.

By the time dad got home, I was numb. I had paced the length of our hallway long enough that I may have worn out the carpet. Nothing made sense that night. I pictured a surgeon standing over her, holding her non-beating heart, and literally squeezing life back into her. That image was equally comforting and terrifying. *Was my mom blessed because they were able to restart her heart or was she cursed because her heart stopped in the first place?* Deep down, I was scared, but at the same time, too confused to be scared. *What was I scared of? She was alive and sleeping. She was comfortable and unaware that she had suffered a surgical complication.* Those were the lies I was telling myself to keep my biggest fears at bay.

Ashley and I just blurted it out the minute he walked through the front door. "Mom had a heart attack," we said in unison. Dad stared blankly for a moment.

"When?" he asked.

"Right after you left. While you were on the train, the hospital called," I told him.

There wasn't much more to say. That was all we knew at that point. We went to sleep and planned on going to see mom the next day. I didn't sleep. Instead, I napped, waking up every few hours. I hadn't felt this helpless and alone since the last time I was the one in the hospital. Growing up, I didn't have many of those nights. Normally mom stayed with me. This is the first I ever felt truly alone. Ashley had Gianna to tend to. Dad had another beer to soothe himself. I was left alone with my thoughts, a mishmash of memories of all the times my mom acted like a warrior.

When she had her jaw broken during a training exercise for the police department, she couldn't eat anything for weeks. She drank all her meals but still made her family dinner every night.

The day drove past a man who had gotten his leg stuck in his car door, she dug out the snow bank, keeping the door closed with her bare hands. I watched from the passenger seat as she pried open his car door. His leg was clearly broken. She asked a stranger in a nearby house to call 911. She then stood outside in the cold holding the door open so it didn't close on his badly damaged leg again.

I remembered how throughout my entire childhood, she was strong for me before I knew how to be strong for myself. *She certainly was strong enough to get through a heart attack, wasn't she? Of course she was.* Besides, she was only 52. That definitely wasn't *old.*

I prayed that night. I've prayed every night since I was a little girl. This was the first night I didn't ask to be given something. I didn't ask to be blessed or protected. I didn't ask that God continue protecting my bones so I wouldn't fracture. I didn't ask Him to send a cure for AIDS or cancer. I didn't ask to land my dream career or to get out of debt. Instead, I asked Him not to take something.

"God, please don't take my mom to heaven yet. She's still very much needed here," I whispered.

I wholeheartedly believed in God. I knew he only had my best interest at heart. I'd experienced God's grace and mercy firsthand. There was no scientific explanation for why, at 29, after being given a life expectancy of 10 years, having a stroke and undergoing open heart surgery, I was still alive. It was God's hand all over my life. I knew if I prayed hard enough and relied on my faith, mom would come through like the warrior I knew her to be.

When we went to the hospital the next day, she didn't look much like a warrior. She was on a ventilator so they had her sedated. She was asleep with her eyes open. I was stunned when I saw her. The night before, the nurse said she was fine and asleep. Nowhere in there did she mention she also wasn't breathing on her own. Nobody warned me she'd be so heavily sedated that she wouldn't know I was there. I wasn't prepared for that first visit. Nobody was. Dad followed my lead. If I moved closer to her bed, so did he. If I took her hand, he felt comfortable doing so. He didn't need permission, but he needed guidance. Dad spent the majority of his adult life having mom tell him where to go, what to say, what to wear, and how to get there. Dad had no clue how to be anybody's advocate. I spent my childhood watching my mother advocate for me. I was 29 and knew how to *fight* insurance companies, doctors who believed in phantom symptoms, and be a fierce advocate to get everything I needed with regard to health care. Essentially, I was a pro at it. When dad felt compelled to look for permission to hold his own wife's hand, I knew mom needed an advocate, and if anyone was designed for the job, it was me.

I declared myself mom's health care proxy. There was no paperwork. The hospital didn't ask any questions. I knew dad wouldn't object. If anything, he was relieved to have someone be the point person and just give him the Cliff Notes version. I knew he didn't really want control. He never even asked me what a health care proxy was. It wasn't a total lie. Mom and I had this conversation years earlier.

I remember that secret pact we made at our kitchen table. She would not leave me on life support and I wouldn't do that to her either, but we wouldn't give up on each other "too early." Looking at her on that ventilator, I had no idea what "too early" looked like. I knew right now looked painful. I looked hard. It looked unfair.

It felt like we were on an out-of-control rollercoaster ride. One day she was getting better, but the next, she would have a stroke. She was still heavily sedated. It was uncertain what she would be like, if she ever woke up after the stroke, or if she could ever recover from it.

Doctors knew she had brain activity because she moved, she moaned, she made sounds trying to speak, and she responded to pain. There was no way to gauge her mental capacity at that point. I worried about the depth of any cognitive dysfunction she may have been left with. She watched her father as his brain was ravaged by Alzheimer's Disease. She was terrified that would be her fate. I was concerned with how she would feel if she woke up and couldn't tie her shoes, remember the names of her children, cook, or hold a job.

Dad and I took the train into the city every day. Ashley stayed home. She had Gianna to take care of. It's not exactly ideal to bring a 9-month-old into any hospital, let alone the ICU. I wish she could have gone more. It was difficult being alone with dad. We spent most of those train rides in complete silence. I wanted to comfort him. I wanted to be hopeful and optimistic. Everyone in my family thought I was "strong." They saw my own medical challenges as proof of my "strength." I wasn't as strong as people thought. I was just unwilling to seem weak in a life that gave me no choice. I could feign strength in every situation except this one. All I could offer up was a half-hearted "She'll be okay." I wasn't sure if I was saying it to reassure dad and Ashley or if I was trying to convince myself that she would be fine. It was as if I said it enough then God would make it true.

Every day I saw her, she looked a little less like my mom. That strength and vigor that radiated out of her body had been reduced to eyes that stared fixated on the ceiling, arms that couldn't hug me, and a voice that couldn't soothe me. Sitting on the outside of the bed was a much different experience than being the patient. *How had she stood on this side of the bed my whole life? How was she able to hold my hand?* My stomach was in knots every time I saw her. I'd ask questions and have to ask doctors to repeat themselves because I could see their lips moving, but I couldn't hear their answers. I was too busy formulating my next question. I'd go home and Google their answers, hoping to find something they missed.

I called up Dr. Loulmet's office and spoke to his assistant. I cried into the phone as I told her what happened to mom and begged that she have Dr. Loulmet call. He had gotten me through heart surgery seamlessly. Of course, he'd have answers. I thought if I could just get him to go to the hospital and work with her team she'd recover. Dr. Loulmet told me he didn't have credentials to work in the hospital that she was in, so he couldn't physically treat her, but he gave me his cellphone number and told me I could call him with any questions I had. If I wanted a second opinion about anything I heard from her team, he was willing to be it. One evening, after a particularly arduous day, I called him.

"He's a good doctor," he said.

I was a bit caught off guard.

"Excuse me?" I asked.

"Her surgeon. I know him. In fact, I know her whole team. She's in good hands."

I'm not sure whether that bolstered my faith in her doctors or shook it. I didn't think I had implied that mom was surrounded by bad doctors. *Was Dr. Loulmet defending them or comforting me?*

It didn't matter. He became my point person. I called Dr. Loulmet with every piece of information I got. Sometimes, I just called him to give him her vitals for that day. He'd tell me what was in a normal range and what wasn't. He coached me on what questions to ask. He kindly gave me his time free of charge. He offered reassurance, but stopped just short of giving me a prognosis. Sometimes he'd say, "That sounds good," or "Sounds like she had a good day." He never said the one thing I wanted to hear: "She's going to be okay." He either didn't want to be responsible for lying to me or her prognosis was legitimately unknown to even a world-renowned cardiothoracic surgeon.

She had good days, and then she'd have a week of bad days. Sometimes we couldn't tell if she was getting better or if she was dying. I'd live for her good days. Those were the days when she'd be somewhat awake and know I was there. Even though her eyes looked hollow, I loved when she would look at me. I'd feel those looks in my soul. I knew she saw me. I held my breath every time she was a little more alert. I was anxiously waiting for doctors to tell me that she could come off the ventilator. I knew it wouldn't be until she was breathing on her own that doctors would be able to ease the sedation enough for her to wake up.

At one point, she was doing so well that we started looking at rehab facilities. I allowed myself to feel hopeful. I thought about all the things we'd do as soon as she was better. I knew she'd fight us on going to rehab. I was looking forward to that fight. I practiced it in my head. I was going to remind her of all the years she made me go to physical therapy when I had no desire to. Ashley spent hours researching alternative healing methods and practices. I prayed a lot. Surely God was going to come through. But I noticed only my family was planning long-term. Her team was just planning for the next day. I thought *this is just medicine.* Doctors have to live in the here and now. Maybe they can't allow themselves to think beyond the immediate. I also knew sometimes I should only plan for this minute because tomorrow is not guaranteed to anyone. No matter how realistic I wanted to be, I had to think long-term. Like mom once told me, "It's now, not forever." I didn't expect this time to last.

We were hopeful. So hopeful that we were caught off guard when her vitals became consistently unstable. Her bad days were not leaving any room for the good days. Her heart function was inadequate, and she could no longer tolerate a reduction in the oxygen flow from the ventilator. Her limbs were turning black. They were dying from the lack of blood flow. The human body is a self-servicing machine. It protects its most vital parts at the expense of others. When the cardiac output is insufficient, the body makes sure blood makes its way to all the organs, often leaving the limbs without any blood flow. Lack of oxygenated blood to any part of the body equals the death of that part.

In an effort to stave off infection, doctors would debride her left hand and both legs. They would force me to stand behind the curtain. I hated that. She would never have left me alone for any procedure. They told me they gave her pain medication before they started, but I could tell she felt it. When I'd come back in, I could see the pain in her eyes. Every time I wanted to leave, or even thought about crying, I remembered, "*She did this for you!*" Every cast, stitch, staple, and surgery, she was right by my side. This woman even shaved my head as I cried my eyes out after my stroke. She never had to look away or walk out. She was my rock. She deserved the same.

"The line of demarcation." If I never hear that term again, it'll be too soon. The line that separates her gangrenous tissues from what little healthy tissue she had left on her limbs. That's what we were waiting for.

When doctors told us that the "best course of action" would be to amputate three of her four limbs, I thought they were crazy. How could cutting off her limbs be best in any scenario? They explained that no amount of recovery time, no miracle, or even if her blood started circulating properly could repair the dead tissue. The muscles, skin, and bone that made up her legs and hand were gone, and nothing was going to bring them back.

"We just need to wait for the line of demarcation." They needed to know exactly how much of her legs and left arm could be salvaged.

Everybody looked at me. I felt the pressure of the question that hung between me, Ashley, and dad. *What should we do?* I was the wrong person to ask. I saw disability through the lens of my life and how I lived it. Being disabled "isn't that bad," I told them. I had a friend who is a quadruple amputee. He's a motivational speaker, and I thought when the time came, I'd just get him to make a special trip from Georgia to New York to speak to her. I naively thought I'd "teach" her how to be disabled. As if there's a textbook for it. I didn't see the situation from her point of view. She was a strong independent woman who lived her life in service to the people she loved. She was not accustomed to relying on other people. I was considering a decision that would make her profoundly disabled. I didn't let myself go there. Doctors said this was the only way to ensure she would not get a deadly infection.

When I weighed death and disability, disability didn't seem that bad. I'd been disabled for 29 years and had a pretty damn good life. In part because mom made sure I had a good life. I could teach her how to push a wheelchair, but I wouldn't be able to teach her how to mourn what she had, what I consciously took away from her. Would she hate me every time she wanted to buy and new pair of heels and remembered she didn't have legs? I wouldn't be able to teach her how to continue making her famous fried chicken or pecan pies with only one hand. So why were they all looking at me? It was because someone had to do it.

"We want her alive. If this keeps her alive, we can worry about the rest later," I told my dad.

"So, you think we should do it?" he asked.

There was no right answer to that question. Of course, I didn't think we should make mom a triple amputee! I was focused on saving her life. Maybe it was selfish, but I wanted her here with me. If it meant that we'd have to sacrifice her legs for her to be here, so be it.

"I think we should do it, dad."

Ashley wasn't thrilled, but she was on board.

We all just wanted to give her the best shot at surviving this catastrophe.

Like any other day, we visited her after surgery. Her legs were amputated above the knee, and her left arm right above the wrist. Heading to the city, I knew I'd see her with no legs. Yet I was still shocked when I walked into the room and saw her stumps wrapped in stark white gauze. That image is forever burned in my mind. I second-guessed everything we were trying to do at that moment. She writhed in the bed. Weeks earlier, they had performed a tracheostomy on her. She no longer had a tube down her throat. The ventilator was now directly connected to a trach tube. This allowed her to try and speak. Even if she wasn't making much noise as she struggled to speak, I understood her. I'd watch her lips move and make out what she was trying to say. It was nothing like the conversations we once had, but it was something to hold on to. Something that gave us hope. She kicked what used to be her legs in the air and moaned in pain.

"Calm down, mom. I'll get the nurse to bring you some meds," I said softly.

She looked at me, eyes dull and teary, and said, "God, what did they do to me?"

I knew that wasn't a complaint as much as a genuine question. Mom spoke to God often and almost always out loud.

I could only imagine what she was going through. I was all too familiar with orthopedic pain. It hurt like hell. There is no other pain like it on this planet. I felt compelled to stay with her. Even though I knew she'd sleep most of the night, I wanted to be with her.

"I want to stay with you tonight," I told her. Dad was standing in the doorway. I knew he could make it back home without me.

"Why don't you?" she said in a faint voice. I was caught off guard that she was alert enough to understand me and respond. I looked at dad and expected him to say we had to go. My heart wanted to stay with her, it really did, but my mind needed a break. Dad just stood there in the doorway.

"I can't, mom." I couldn't because I was terrified and I felt incredibly guilty. I knew I didn't have it in me to watch her in pain all night. She fell back asleep and didn't question me further.

To this day, I hate myself for that. I couldn't stay because I was tired. I was hungry and I was emotionally exhausted. I was selfish. I had forgotten about all the times she slept in a chair by my bedside to be the first person I saw when I woke up. She did everything in her power to ensure I never felt alone. For one night, I couldn't do that for her. I'll regret that for the rest of my life.

I worried that mom's pain would go uncontrolled and she'd be unable to ask for pain medication. With my mom sedated, I didn't trust that they would give her painkillers every six to eight hours as recommended. I needed to hate myself less for leaving so I was going to make sure I took care of that before I left. I asked her nurse what was prescribed for pain. She told me that she had an order for intravenous morphine.

"If it's called for every six to eight hours, do not let her go more than seven hours without it," I said firmly.

The nurse looked at me. She was cold. Maybe I was just stressed and tired, but I did not like her.

"I understand you're concerned, but I know how to do my job," she said.

I didn't doubt she knew how to do her job. I doubted that she knew how to care for my mom and I was making no apologies for that.

"This is not about your job! That's my mom!" I told her.

She nodded. I felt good enough that I had made my point.

"Yes, and my job is to care for your mom tonight so you can get some rest."

I knew I was being dismissed but was too tired to get upset about it. After that, I ran into mom's room and told her that I had spoken to the nurse and she would have all the pain control she needed. I told her I loved her and that I would see her the next day.

Each day, it became a little harder to see her. I wanted to see her. I wanted to talk to her, but every day it felt like it was just more bad news. Every day she looked a little less like herself. She'd lost so much weight. Her kidneys were failing so she was getting dialysis, which made her face puffy, but everything else was so gaunt. I hoped. I prayed. Consciously I wanted her to be okay. Subconsciously I wanted her to be at peace. At the moment, I didn't know what peace would be, but I knew it wasn't this. I wasn't 100 percent sure what was on the other side, yet I knew that a merciful God, the one she raised me to believe in, wouldn't want this for her. I knew she was suffering. Whenever I was in the hospital, mom would tell me, "When your child is in pain, you feel it in your soul because you feel that pain too."

Now I understood what she meant by that. It's this visceral ache deep inside that just lingers. You don't even know what hurts, but you know that something is definitely in pain. I was helpless. The only thing I could do was pray. God, I prayed. I prayed harder than I'd ever prayed before. I grabbed my rosary at night and tried to pray with it. I kept forgetting the order. *Was Our Father first? How many times were you supposed to say Hail Mary?* Mom taught me how to pray with the rosary before my first Holy Communion. I am certain that God didn't know what the hell I was doing right now. So I went back to asking for my mom to live.

"God, please don't take her to Heaven yet," I pleaded.

I'd be lying if I said I was relieved when doctors talked to us about this being the end. Despite their best efforts and the amputations, mom still developed an infection. I don't think anyone was surprised by that. She had been in the hospital for three months. The quickest way to get an infection is to spend a significant amount of time in the hospital. She had sepsis and had entered multi-organ failure.

"Dying with dignity," they called it.

She was on the ventilator so she was only technically alive. It would be relatively easy. They would increase her sedation and disconnect her ventilator. Within a few minutes, she'd pass away peacefully without ever waking from the sedation. *Did they really just say dignity? What was dignified about cutting off her limbs? What was dignified about the hole they cut in her throat? What was dignified about the strongest person I knew being reduced to a shell of herself?*

I thought back to that conversation we had months ago. "Promise you'll do the same for me," she said. I didn't know nor could I prove where she was, but I was certain she was not in that bed. I had prayed to God to help me, to help her find peace. The answer wasn't in my millionth Google search. It wasn't in my next conversation with Dr. Loulmet. The answer to her finding the peace she deserved was in letting her go, letting her be with the God she so believed in.

Shortly before mom scheduled her surgery, grandma was diagnosed with throat cancer. While I was consumed with mom and her health care, grandma passed away. I like to believe that all the times I saw mom staring at the ceiling she was actually looking at grandma.

I desperately wanted dad to come to me and say, "We're taking your mom off life support." I wanted it to be his decision. I would have backed him, but I wanted him to feel in control. *Who was I kidding?* The last thing dad ever wanted was control. He was content having every decision made for him. Mom decided everything from the dinner menu to how they would raise their children. There was no "Go ask your father" in my house. Mom called the shots and dad complied. To ask him to make a literal life or death decision was almost cruel. I took him out into the hall. I didn't want to risk mom hearing what I was about to say. She was probably already out of her body but I didn't want her to know she was about to die.

I took dad's hand. I can't remember the last time we touched. The last time we were in such close proximity was the day his mom, Nana, died. Something about death always seemed to draw us close.

"We can't do this to her anymore," I told him.

He took a few deep breaths but didn't say anything.

You're going to make me tell you that it's okay to kill her, aren't you?

Early that morning, I had a conversation with mom's nurse, Peck. He was the nicest guy in that whole hospital. I asked him for guidance. I asked him what he would do if this was his mom.

"I wouldn't leave my mom like this," he said. "You know she's not living. She's just alive. You know the difference. They can keep her alive as long as you want, but she'll never live again. That's not fair to her."

That resonated deeply within my soul. Mom would not want to just "be alive." She wanted to live. She had a whole list of things she wanted to do in retirement. She wanted to travel. She wanted to run her own financial services business. She had recently passed her series six and 67 securities exams. Whether we kept her alive on not, her life would stop at 52.

"We can't be selfish, dad," I said.

"I know, we can't," he replied.

The truth is, I wanted to be incredibly selfish. I wanted to keep her on this planet and keep praying for miracles. One day, God would hear me and she would have a miraculous recovery. My heart said that's not reality. My heart said, "This woman sacrificed everything for you and your sister. In this moment, you have to be selfless. She spent 29 years of your life being the example of selflessness!" I knew there was no decision to be made. I just had to be courageous enough to say it.

"Dad, let's let her go. We have to."

He agreed. "We have to. Call your sister."

That's easily the hardest phone call I've ever had to make.

"Ashley, get here as soon as you can. We're going to take mom off life support." I needed to say that because it made it real.

It was no longer this ambiguous idea. My mom was going to die that night.

I sat with her and rubbed her hand. I tried to disguise my tension and fear. If she was anywhere in that room, even if not in her body, she felt my fear. I was absolutely terrified to live the rest of my life without her. I knew Ashley had a 90-minute train ride and we weren't going to do this without her, so I knew I had at least an hour and a half.

I whispered, "I love you." A whisper felt more natural than my full voice in this moment. The room felt so clean, dull, and sterile. I don't remember it being this cold in here during any of our visits. If Heaven is as bright and vibrant in color as mom told me, she was in for a shock.

One night, we watched the Robin Williams movie *What Dreams May Come.* "That's what Heaven looks like, Taniya," she said. Whatever it looked like, it certainly didn't look like this room. I told her how proud I was of her. My mind raced to think of things that didn't sound cliche. No one tells you how to say goodbye forever.

These are the last things you'll ever say to her. Don't regret it.

The words "thank you" were inadequate.

How many times had I been on the other side of this bed? How many times did she sit stoically holding my hand?

I wished she could have explained to me how she did that part or the rules of how it was supposed to work. My stomach didn't feel well. I was somewhere between being hungry and wanting to throw up.

"You put up a good fight. I know you're tired," I said finally.

I'm not 100% sure what I meant by that, but it sounded like something she would say to me if the roles were reversed. The beeping monitors seemed so loud all of a sudden.

"It's okay," dad said every time he noticed that sound.

I don't know if he was talking to himself, me, or mom. It didn't matter because it was nice to hear something besides the damn beeping. I still couldn't speak above a whisper. When I took my eyes off her, I looked at the clock on the wall. The hands were moving, but time felt like it was standing still. I'm not sure which was harder to look at.

When Ashley arrived, it felt like time stopped and sped up simultaneously. I second-guessed if we were making the right decision, but I knew I had to remain strong and stoic. I was never afforded the luxury of falling apart. As early as I can remember, I was praised for being "strong." I held on to all my stress, fear, and pain in silence. I knew if I cracked, dad would leave her on life support until he died. He asked me at least three times, "Are you okay?" I knew that was my cue to say, "No! Let's not do this." But I responded the same way each time, teary eyed. "Yea, I'm okay. We're going to be okay." It didn't make sense that any of us would be okay without her, but I said it with conviction.

The nurse came in with paperwork for dad to sign. I shook my head. Hearing is the last sense to go when you die. Mom could still hear. I didn't want the very last thing she heard in her life to be hearing her death being planned.

"Take that in the hall," I requested.

The nurse left and we all followed. Dad signed all the consent forms and I felt like I was going to throw up. The nurse walked us through the process. She detailed every step with such precision that I could tell this wasn't the first time she'd done this. We were not the first family to remove their loved one from life support. The thought that *other people do this* was oddly comforting. Then it hit me. *We are not terrible people.* I needed to sit with that thought for a minute. I think I tuned out most of what she said. I was thinking about how could I possibly get out of bed in the morning knowing I was instrumental in killing my mother. I felt the weight of that like no other pressure I've ever felt before. I asked the nurse to promise me that mom would not know and she wouldn't feel anything. I worried she would struggle to breathe. Would she feel herself suffocating? If her death was imminent, it had to be peaceful. We had put her through more than any one person should endure. I wanted to guarantee her a few moments of peace before she left this world. My whole life, she was my soft place to fall. She deserved similar comfort.

"She won't know or feel anything. Nothing will happen until I know she is deeply asleep. She'll fall asleep, and she just won't wake up. She will have no pain or fear," the nurse said.

Her answer felt honest and sincere. She made me comfortable. As comfortable as you can be knowing your mother, best friend, confidant, and biggest cheerleader was about to die in front of you.

I climbed into bed with her. I curled up next to her as they injected the sedation into her IV. Ashley sat on the other side. Mom laid there flanked by the two grown women she once gave birth to. We spoke in hushed voices, as if she really were sleeping and we didn't want to disturb her. We all knew it was deeper than the average nighttime sleep. She was way deeper than REM, but there was a respect we always had for mom when she slept. That dates back to her years at the police department. She worked from 11 p.m. until 7 a.m. She'd get a few hours of sleep between getting us on the school bus and us coming home. She may have gotten a few more hours between homework and having to start dinner. Her sleep was precious because she didn't get much. Ashley and I always tried to be as quiet as a church mouse and only wake her for really pressing issues. However, when you're a little kid, a really pressing issue is whether or not you can open the new bag of Cheetos, so we woke her up often and, sometimes, obnoxiously.

She was about to catch up on all her missed sleep. The nurse came in without making much noise. It was as if she respected the sanctity of this space in that moment. These were the last few minutes of my mom's life. It was more than just reminiscing on a life well lived. It was worshiping a woman who pledged her love and devoted her life to all three of us. This was a woman who lived a life of service without ever trying. That was just who she was. She weaved a complex story of sacrifice and pure love.

"I had a great life," she said on many occasions when talking about being a young mom and the mother of a disabled child. In spite of everything I saw her give up and endure in her life, she still thought it was great. I hoped in this moment she knew my life was great too, solely because she made it so. I wondered how my life could continue to be great without her.

The next time the nurse came, it felt different. Her warm demeanor and light step was replaced by a laser beam focus and heaviness. I didn't like the way that felt. At the same time, I felt compassion for her. None of us wanted to be here right now. She had been mom's nurse for several weeks. She would end a life momentarily. I wondered if she learned in nursing school how to do this. I couldn't imagine this as a lesson in a textbook. *Did she feel as guilty as I did right now?* I knew her entrance signaled the end. It was hard to comprehend how we got here.

In reality, this moment was three months in the making. My mom spent three months in the ICU, never really recovering and never waking up for any considerable length of time. She never got to enjoy hitting all the milestones on the road to recovery like I had. It all seemed so unfair, and I felt guilty. The nurse disconnected the hose that connected mom's trach tube to the ventilator. Despite the colloquial term to "pull the plug," there was no plug to pull. Taking someone off life support has nothing to do with the power that runs the machine. I heard the ventilator still running in the background, but the connection between that and mom had been severed.

I stared up at the monitor that had tracked her vitals for three months. I saw the space that always displayed her pulse drop quickly until numbers were no longer present. Instead, it just displayed two empty dashes. There was no rise and fall of her chest anymore. Even though it had been mechanical, I noticed when her lungs filled with the oxygen forced in by the ventilator. I prayed in my head. I silently asked God to welcome her into Heaven and ease any trepidation she may have upon arriving. I was startled out of my moment of prayer by the ear-numbing monotone beep the monitor made when her heart stopped. I looked up to see the flat, solid red line with no peaks or valleys. I used to watch those peaks and valleys, hoping to eventually see a consistent rhythm. That was never to be.

I felt it the minute her soul left her body. The energy in the room changed. It was a dynamic shift as if everything that was her was sucked out of that room. The air felt thick. The calm that her presence brought was gone. I felt more tranquil and calm watching her die than I did in the moments after she left this world.

A faint voice in the distance announced the time. I knew they were calling her time of death. Time was irrelevant right now. Mom was gone. Unless we could rewind three months, I didn't care what time it was. I threw myself onto her body and sobbed. The only thing I could think to say was, "I'm sorry!" I felt like I had failed her, not just in this moment, but in life.

"I will make you proud, mom! I will find a way to make you proud!" I repeated over and over.

I was grieving. I was mourning, but I was also listening for a heartbeat. I remembered when she had asked me, "How do they know you're dead before they bury you?" I saw all the fields on the monitor go blank. She was pronounced dead. But what if she had some premonition when she asked me that? I had to hear with my own ears that her heart had stopped.

Ashley grabbed me by my shoulders and pulled me up.

"You already made her proud," she told me.

Had I? Nothing in me felt like I'd done anything to make her proud. She had big dreams for me. When I'd ask her where my name came from, she'd proudly say, "I made it up! I liked the way it looked. I could see it on a business card, office door plaque, or lab coat." I hadn't lived up to any of that. And now she wasn't here to see whatever I may have become. If I had never felt like a failure before, I did in that moment.

The three of us left the hospital for the last time that night. I knew I'd never have to see my mom in that type of pain ever again. I also knew I'd never see my mom ever again. We were tired and emotionally battered. I expected that because we knew she was going to die, it would hurt less. We essentially planned it. It didn't catch us off guard. So why did my heart feel like it had been ripped out of my chest and destroyed?

We took the train home. It was a Thursday night, one day before the 4th of July. It was a big party night in the city. A group of rowdy boys got on the train. They were loud and clearly intoxicated. On a normal night, I'd only find drunk boys slightly irritating. Not this night. They enraged me. If I was not physically and emotionally exhausted, I might have screamed, "Shut the hell up!" I wasn't mad at them. I was mad that they were happy. Why did they get to be happy? Didn't they realize what the world had just lost? They didn't know Deborah Faulk. They'd never even heard of her. They had no obligation to mourn her death. I hated that because I just wanted the world to stop. I wanted no one to be happy until I wasn't in this much pain.

I was raised Roman Catholic. Mom deeply believed in God and that God had a plan. One of the tenants of our house was, "Do not question God, just trust his plan." In the moment she died, I couldn't help but question God. *What made me worthy of miracles?* I was a dumb 29-year-old. I hadn't sacrificed very much or contributed to this world in any significant way. My life had been spared multiple times. Why? What did God believe I had that would add anything to this world? Whatever it was, I'd never live up to it. Especially without mom, my entire support system, by my side.

So I'll Go...

Whitney Houston was Mom's favorite singer. When she finally had her own home, mom declared every Sunday to be "Cleaning Sunday." She'd put on a Whitney CD and dance around while bleaching, scrubbing, and vacuuming. She moved differently when Whitney's music was on. Her favorite song was "I Will Always Love You." She sang it all the time. It never got old. Mom had a beautiful voice. If I close my eyes, I can still hear her singing it. Immediately after her death, I heard that song differently. It was no longer just a chart-topper. It was prophecy. Two lines, specifically, stood out: "If I should stay, I would only be in your way. So I'll go but I know I'll think of you every step of the way."

I found comfort in believing that her death was her final act of selflessness. She was now a triple amputee. No matter how well I thought I could teach her to be disabled, I didn't know how to teach anyone how to be independent. I was still learning that myself. What if her biggest fear came true? What if she did get Alzheimer's Disease? Who would she be able to rely on? She would have felt like a burden. As someone who dedicated her life to caring for others, she wouldn't have transitioned well into a person requiring care. Maybe that was just a whimsical thought that made me feel better at the time. I had to believe that she died on her terms, and not that God just ripped her away from people who loved her dearly. That's a thought I feel deep in my soul to this day.

"We both know I'm not what you need." If she could speak, those would have been her last words to me. She worked so hard to make sure I could make it in life without her.

Maybe I didn't *need* her, but God knows I wanted her. I was deeply depressed. I felt guilty as hell. I had survivor's guilt. How had we had the same surgery with drastically different outcomes? She didn't deserve what she got. *I was sick my whole life.* I'd cheated death before. God had shown me so much grace throughout my life. He spared me when I should have died. Her life was so much more impactful than mine. Why didn't he save her? If she was going to die, why didn't he just take her? Why did she have to suffer? Above all, why did I have to make the decision to end her life when she spent her entire life advocating for and trying to save mine? It felt like a cruel joke.

Almost immediately my faith in God waned. I'd never questioned God. I was raised not to. Every challenge, injury, and pain I endured, I never asked, "Why me?" I accepted this as my life. All of it was par for the course. My faith had remained unshaken through it all. Until now. I wasn't asking, "Why me?" I was asking, "Why her?" I couldn't reconcile the idea of a merciful all-loving God and the three months of hell He just made her endure. I gave up on the idea that God has a plan. Suddenly, everything I was taught didn't make sense. Plans have a point. My mom's death seemed senseless. I held tight to my belief in Heaven because I had to believe that she was somewhere. She was in a place I could easily get to if I really wanted to. I slowly started wanting to die. Not because of life, but because I believe the minute I'm not on this planet, I'll be with her. At that point, there was nothing I wanted more than to be reunited with her.

If there was any plan or miracle to be found in this pain, it was Gianna. In what felt like an act of divine timing, there she was: a new life that entered our family one year before mom passed away. When Ashley announced she was pregnant, it made no sense. Ashley was young, single, and living with her parents. But God had a plan.

Three-hundred and sixty-four days after Gianna was born, we watched our mother pass away. Gianna was the physical manifestation of *the circle of life.* Twenty-four hours from that day, she turned 1 year old. She deserved to be celebrated. God bless Ashley, who stayed up planning for a small party. I went to sleep praying not to wake up in the morning. I think Ashley needed to stay busy that first night. It wasn't just the first night, and it wasn't just Ashley who needed to be busy. Gianna was the glue that held us all together. She definitely saved my life.

I was consumed by my grief. I was afraid. I was alone. I was in tremendous pain. I'd wake up mad at God nearly every day. I couldn't shake the horrific images of mom's lifeless body in that hospital bed. I wanted to imagine her dancing in Heaven, but when I closed my eyes, all I could see was her in a casket, cold, alone and underground. I'd thought if I died right now, dad could bury me in the double plot he bought for her and we could be together again. It bothered me that she was alone. I believed in Heaven and I knew her soul was not underground, but my mind was stuck on the idea of her physical body.

In my darkest moments, I'd look in my dresser drawer and see every bottle of opioids I'd ever been prescribed. I hated taking opioids. I didn't like the way they made me feel and didn't want to become addicted. I was also afraid to throw them out. What if I suffered a really bad fracture and needed serious pain relief? I kept them away in my top dresser drawer. Three bottles of Vicodin, a bottle of Oxycodone, and enough Ambien to sleep for a decade. I also had my anti-epileptic drugs and all the Prozac I've ever been prescribed. I'd look around and wonder how many of each, or what combination, would allow me to end it all. I was in a super scary place. After everything I endured, this was the moment I wanted to die. I didn't believe in God anymore, which I couldn't reconcile because I still believed in Heaven.

Every morning I'd walk out of my room and go into the living room to see Gianna. She'd smile and squeal as soon as she saw me. She was love in its purest form. She called me *Ah-Iya*. Her version of Aunt Taniya, which certainly is a mouth full. I couldn't look at this perfect little baby and not believe in God. People are born and people die every day. God's hand is in both. Seeing life through the eyes of a toddler and experiencing everything for the first time was enough to solidify one's belief in God. They are a reminder that life does go on and that life is pretty incredible. If I could feel Gianna's joy as much as I felt my grief, I could remember there's a reason I'm here. Mom hadn't spent 29 years fighting for me for no reason. She never gave up on me. She would be so disappointed if I gave up on myself.

I'd look at Gianna and know I was exactly where I needed to be and didn't have the right to disrupt that. Ashley was a single mom without a mother anymore. Down the road, she may need support. Gianna deserved as many people as possible to love her. The joy she bought slowly eased my grief. The anger I felt towards God for taking my mom was replaced with gratitude. I was deeply grateful for Gianna's presence. I was grateful that she was on this Earth and I was grateful every time she reached for me. She was the embodiment of all that is right in this world. She needed me to stay. If not for her, I'm not convinced I'd still be here. She restored my faith in God and she filled the worst time of my life with happiness. She was the light when I could only see darkness. She'll seek purpose as she grows older, but I'm certain part of her purpose was to give me, Ashley, and dad a reason to want to go on.

Haywire

After Mom died, my seizures got worse. I couldn't go a day without seizing, sometimes multiple times a day. Every time I had another seizure, my neurologist changed my medication or increased the dosage. Anti-epileptic drugs are not kind. They come with a series of side effects, and I seemed to experience all of them throughout the course of treatment: dizziness, headaches, insomnia, intense dreams, depression, anxiety, and mood swings. At the height of my epilepsy, I was on 4,800 milligrams of AEDs and still had seizures. They were seemingly uncontrollable. I took my medication religiously and still couldn't find peace.

It's hard to describe what a seizure feels like to someone who has never had one. I'd feel it coming on. The left side of my face would tingle or go numb completely, and I'd get a strange taste in my mouth. It tasted like I was sucking on mint-flavored metal. That would be my sign that my brain was about to be taken over. I'd stay aware but have no control of my body or my mind. Once, I was walking through a store and felt a seizure coming on. I knew I shouldn't be standing while having a seizure. The risk of falling and breaking something was too great. I sat down and leaned up against a wall. I was going to let the seizure pass and go on with my day. The minute the seizure started, I began to bang my head against the wall. I could feel the pain and was conscious enough to think to myself, "S*top banging your head. You're going to give yourself another brain injury or crack your skull.*" I was processing rational thoughts but had no ability to make my body respond. After any seizure ended, I would be left with no energy. My muscles would ache and I would need to sleep for hours to regain any semblance of myself.

If there was such a thing as a good seizure, it would be the ones I had in my sleep. My mom would visit me during those. They aren't dreams because I could feel myself open my eyes. I'd have all my typical seizure hallucinations: glowing orbs in various colors floating in space. I'd see my mom standing among them. Consciously I'd try to sit up so I could hug her, but I couldn't move. I'd want to call out to her, but I couldn't formulate any words or make any sounds. So I'd just stare at her until it was over. I'd wake up and only know I had a seizure because all of the things on my nightstand would be knocked over, and I'd feel like I hadn't slept in a week. I told my doctor about my nocturnal seizures, hoping he'd validate with some metaphysical reasoning. I wanted to hear something along the lines of, "Many patients report going to Heaven or seeing deceased loved ones." I don't know what made me think I could get that from a man who dedicated his life to neuroscience. Instead, what I got was a very rational and physical explanation.

"Most memories are stored in your temporal lobe, the exact place your seizures originate from. You're experiencing heightened autobiographical memories incited by the increased neurological synapses and activity." That was a perfectly scientific answer.

I didn't believe it then, and I still don't believe it now. My mom used my nocturnal seizures as an opportunity to let me know she hadn't left me.

The seizures I had while I was awake started to include strange hallucinations. I saw my dog talk. I saw a rainbow. It felt oddly familiar. I talked about it with my neurologist. He reviewed all medical records from the time of the stroke to the present day. He concluded that the car accident I had in 2005 was most likely perpetuated by a seizure. That explained the purple house I saw and the elephant that was crossing the street. They were not random hallucinations. I was having a seizure. My brain was not being deprived of oxygen because of a leaky heart valve. I was having a seizure! That was like a punch to the gut. That original diagnosis led me to have open heart surgery. A surgery that was the catalyst for my mother's death. If not for that misdiagnosis, my mitral valve would still be leaking and my mom might still be alive. She only committed to that surgery because I had it. I'm not convinced she would have started thinking about heart surgery. Perhaps she would have just moved through life, dealing with an occasional angina attack. Maybe she could still be adding beauty and joy to this world, touching people with her light. I may always wonder about that.

I battled uncontrolled epilepsy for another six years. My neurologist at the time was at a loss. We had tried almost every AED on the market in various combinations. Nothing helped. The DMV caught wind of my diagnosis and suspended my license. An "administrative suspension," they called it. I guess that was code for, "You didn't do anything wrong, but we don't trust you on the road." That was humiliating. I was 30 and couldn't drive myself anymore. I hadn't felt that helpless since I was a kid, unable to take myself to the bathroom. The rules were that I had to go 12 months without any seizures, get a doctor to certify that I was seizure-free, and I would be given my license back. That was easier said than done. I couldn't go 12 days without a seizure. I was lucky if I got 12 hours. The DMV stipulation seemed impossible. I felt like there was no hope I'd ever be seizure-free. That held too many limitations.

Long Island is not known for its public transportation. Without driving, how could I hold a job? Forget about having a social life. I had worked too hard to be a functioning adult, and it felt like all that hard work meant nothing. My independence was being stolen from me. As immature as it sounded, all I could think was, "This isn't fair!" I complied because I had to, but I hated it.

My neurologist finally referred me to a neurosurgeon. "You might be a candidate for epilepsy surgery," he said.

Epilepsy surgery? There's such a thing? If there is, why didn't we discuss this six years earlier?

I met the doctor who would become my surgeon in the spring of 2012. Surgery sounded anything but simple. It would be done in two stages. First, he'd perform a full craniotomy. He'd open the right side of my skull and meticulously cut away all the scarred parts of my brain. Most of that was dead and non-functional. Besides the obvious risk of death, it carried little risk that my faculties would be compromised. A few months later, he'd go back in with a stereotactic laser and perform an ablation, or "burn" sections that required more precision. As a surgeon, he had an 85 percent success rate of leaving his patients seizure-free. That was all I needed to hear.

That summer, I underwent surgery. Some friends and family thought I was crazy. Who has elective neurosurgery? I wasn't crazy. I was desperate. I wanted my life back. I hated the uncertainty of having a seizure. It wasn't a matter of *if* I had a seizure anymore. It was *where* I would be when I had one.

I came out of surgery fine. It was a waiting game to see if I had a seizure. The only way to prove the surgery had been successful was to not have a seizure. Every seizure-free day was a reason to celebrate. One day turned into two. Two days turned into three. Before I knew it, I was celebrating months and not days. I went a full year seizure-free. I was so happy and grateful. Mom always said, "When you overcome a challenge, you feel lighter because the weight of that burden has been lifted." I felt light as a feather. I felt unstoppable. Unfortunately, that feeling was short-lived.

After being seizure-free for more than a year, they returned. They didn't just quietly come back. They came back with a vengeance. They were more frequent and worse than before. I was pissed. What happened to my surgeon's 85 percent success rate? I'd watched every interview he gave, looked up all his credentials, and read patient testimonials. Everything was positive. One patient after another talked about their newfound seizure freedom. Why wasn't I part of this exclusive club? I confronted my surgeon about it. Why was I only successful for a year? I wanted a seizure-free lifetime! He told me he was slightly conservative in his original approach.

"You had so much scar tissue near very sensitive parts of your brain," he said. He left some of it in place to preserve my memory and the vision in my left eye.

He offered to schedule a third surgery and remove the last of it. He explained that this one was riskier. He'd be operating in the hippocampus, where the human brain stores all its long-term memories. There was a slight possibility that I'd wake with no memory. I was worried. *What if I woke up and couldn't remember my mom?* Those memories were precious. I didn't fear death because I knew if that was the result, at the very least, she and I would be together. I was terrified of waking up from surgery and having no recollection of who she was and all the amazing things she did for me. I thought quickly about all the surgeries she consented to me having with the promise of making my future better. That's what she wanted for me. With this thought, I was on board.

"Let's go for it," I said to my surgeon. The benefits outweighed the risk.

He scheduled the surgery for the middle of February 2014. Initially, I agreed, until I remembered I had tickets to see Justin

Timberlake in concert at Madison Square Garden two days after the surgery. I knew there was no way I was going to be out of the hospital and strong enough to take the train and walk through NYC. Not to mention that brain surgery left me with a pretty bad headache. Even if I could physically go, it may not be enjoyable. Out of all the risks I was willing to take, missing Justin Timberlake in concert was not one of them. I told my surgeon we had to reschedule my surgery date. He asked why. I told him that I had a concert a few days after my surgery date. He looked at me, perplexed.

"You want to reschedule your surgery for a concert?" He laughed.

"It's not just any concert. It's a *Justin Timberlake* concert! And yes, we will reschedule the surgery."

He pulled out his phone and opened his calendar. "The only day I have available until summer is February 24th."

I told him to book it. That was a week after the concert, so we were in the clear.

I was excited. I felt deep in my soul that this was it. I had the right surgeon and this was going to be a success. I'm not sure who was more determined for it to be a success, me or my surgeon.

I woke up on February 24th, 2014, in room 224. The significance was not lost on me. I knew the synchronicity of the 224 meant something. I felt God's hand all over that day. That brought a sense of peace and a feeling of certainty that I had never felt after any surgery. Normally I pray and hope that recovery goes smoothly. Having the date change made me feel like this was the time and the place that this was supposed to happen. This is what divine timing looks like.

I quickly tried to remember as much as I could to ensure my memory hadn't been destroyed. I was flooded with so many beautiful memories. I could remember the Christmas of 1991 when Mom made her first cheesecake. I could remember the pear tree I climbed. I could remember mom on cleaning Sundays. I could remember every holiday we spent together. It was all still there and I was beyond relieved.

I reflect back on my decision to have that surgery, and I sometimes wonder if I was a bit crazy. Desperation will make you take some bizarre risks. I just wanted my life back. Seven years later, I know it was the best decision I've ever made. It was a decision born of desperation but fueled by courage and faith.

Every year I celebrate two birthdays: July 21st — the day Deborah Faulk gave me life — and February 24th — the day I was given my life back. That's not a day I take lightly. Every year I take the day off from work. I don't schedule anything. I don't do anything that moves me from a place of gratitude. I sit still and thank God for all I've been through and all I've been spared. For me, it's still the most important day on the calendar. When you can look at your life and recognize the moments you almost lost it all, that's a different level of gratitude. It's the closest I've ever come to having a spiritual experience.

Hope + Faith = Perseverance

Often people look at me and compliment my *perseverance.* They call me *determined.* If they only knew how many times I wanted to give up, maybe they wouldn't be so impressed. I am optimistic by nature, but there were things that were hard. Things that I felt I wasn't cut out for. I *hoped* I would walk. I *hoped* people would believe in me. I *hoped* I would recover from my stroke. I *hoped* that I wouldn't grieve my Mom's death for the rest of my life. Optimism wanes as things get harder, even though I was trying my very best. I know they say that God will never give you more than you can handle. Sometimes I wanted to turn to God and say, "I'm not this strong!" More times than I can count, I was ready to throw my hands up in defeat. I told God, "I've fought the good fight. With every struggle you threw at me, I rose to the occasion. What more can you possibly want from me?"

That was a rhetorical question without any answers. Yet, I believed. I believed in something bigger than myself. In moments when I was too tired to *hope* anymore, I fell back on my *faith.* It wasn't perseverance. It was blind, sometimes stupid, *faith.* When I had nothing else, I had my *faith*.

Hope is a transient desire. It's a wish. *Faith* is belief and it is rooted in something much deeper than just what you want to happen. My *faith* has been tested, it's even been shaken to its core. I've been mad at God. I've struggled to find the blessing in the burden. Like my mom always said, God has a plan. It was a crazy, chaotic plan, and I don't know why he planned it for me, but he did.

I can't deny that I've been incredibly blessed. There were many times when things didn't have to work out the way I hoped, but they did. They still do. I know I'm given the credit because I'm who people see. I am the tangible. They see and believe in my courage. They believed in the concept of me overcoming insurmountable obstacles. They held tightly to the image of the "fragile" little girl in a wheelchair determined to walk, determined to go to college, determined to be the best she could be. What they never noticed was the intangible — the silent prayers and the faith that I wouldn't fail because God wouldn't let me. Without my deep-seated faith, my innate fear of failure would have consumed me. I had to be more faithful than I was fearful in order to give what people called "perseverance."

The name of my disease, Osteogenesis Imperfecta, can be broken down to literally mean "imperfect from the beginning." Genesis or formation. Imperfecta or imperfect. I am genetically designed to break. The beauty in that is that no matter how many times I broke a bone, they were designed not to *fall apart.* My life, with all its imperfections, has been the perfect life for me. It has been challenging for sure, but I wouldn't want it any other way. Anyone's life only makes sense when you look at it after it's been lived.

The easiest question one can ask is, "Why me?" Aside from having a self-indulgent moment of pity, you'll never find the answer. It doesn't serve you to ask. If not you, then who? If not now, then when? If not here, then where? There will never be a life devoid of challenges. There will never be a perfect time or a perfect place. You'll never be a perfect person. Sometimes the best we can do is embrace all our broken parts until the cracks mend and we are stronger than before.

It's okay to crack. It's even okay to break. It's inevitable that you'll have moments where you feel it's impossible to keep moving forward, but do it anyway. Much like bones, no matter how hurt, weak, damaged, or broken you may feel, you weren't designed to *fall apart.*

Acknowledgments

God, all things are possible through you. You've sent some of the most amazing doctors, nurses, and therapists my way. I was blessed with some doctors who saw possibilities where others saw "problems." You also surrounded me with the most amazing tribe who made this story easier to live and empowering to tell.

Mom, this story was yours long before it was mine. Everything I am is because of who you were. Your "No bubble wrap" philosophy allowed me to be just as fearless as you were. No words will ever express the depth of my gratitude for your strength and sacrifice. I hope that I make you proud.

Dad, "Tee, you can do anything you set your mind to," still echoes in my ears. A daily reminder I didn't know I needed. I love you.

Ashley, my baby sister, you were literally my "legs" when we were kids and my first best friend. I wouldn't have wanted to walk through life without you by my side. I love you.

Gianna, you were my test audience for much of this book. Your feedback has been invaluable. You are a force that will light up the world one day. Don't ever dull your sparkle because others don't know how to shine. I love you!

Mia, you kept me on my toes. The innocence of your heart and the beauty in your questions kept me on track. Keep dreaming big, little girl. I love you!

Alex, I would never get through life without you. God knew I needed another sister, so he sent you. I am so grateful for you!

Kyle, thank you for just being who you are in my life. Your encouragement and belief in me and my story pushed me to bring this book to fruition. If not for you, this would still be an unfinished file on my MacBook. Your words still inspire me today as much as they did in 2007. I love you!

Keith, you saw what was in my head and translated that into "perfect" imagery.

Anyone who loved and cared for me when it wasn't easy, your love, prayers, and belief in me brightened some of my darkest days.

Made in the USA
Monee, IL
04 November 2026

67387313R10108